The Sociology of South Asian Women's Health

Sara Rizvi Jafree
Editor

The Sociology of South Asian Women's Health

Springer

Editor
Sara Rizvi Jafree
Department of Sociology
Forman Christian College University
Lahore, Pakistan

ISBN 978-3-030-50203-4 ISBN 978-3-030-50204-1 (eBook)
https://doi.org/10.1007/978-3-030-50204-1

This Springer imprint is published by the registered company Springer Nature Switzerland AG
The registered company address is: Gewerbestrasse 11, 6330 Cham, Switzerland

To my Grandmothers:
Syeda Laila Rezvi
Sabiha Shah
Syeda Sikandar Rizvi

Acknowledgments

This book is truly a labor of love and emotions. During the period of researching for the book and writing it, both my parents suffered through cancer. It is true that words are never enough to thank ones parents for their love and sacrifices. Their determined strength to fight for a cure and their faith in God will always be a life lesson for me. Ironically, one of the aims of this book was to highlight the role of self and society in health recovery, and I have learnt firsthand what the meaning of family support is, not just for the sick but also for family attendants and care providers. My other pillars of strength whom I am eternally grateful include my wonderful husband, Baqir, and my amazing daughters, Aliza and Alina.

I would also like to thank all my aunts—my Phupos (Rehana Asad and Khadija Mohib), my Chachi's (Angelina Rezvi and Sayeda Rezvi), and my Mami (Merzieh Shah)—for being consistent role models of fiercely strong, resilient, and loyal women, who inspire me every day to be a better person. I want to take this opportunity to also thank my other Phupos—Noori Mama, Sajjadi Phupo, Ruqaiya Phupo, Narjis Phupo, and Chamki Phupo. I have absorbed the values and ethics that I have seen you practice as a child during long hours of Majalis, and I believe I would not have the faith I have if it were not for all of you.

Many of my co-authors have been with me in different stages of my life, during secondary school in Kuwait and while I was a university student in London. I am so deeply grateful to have worked on this book with some of my oldest friends—Baj, Fareen, Deepti, and Fi. We have seen each other grow during our teenage years, while living in dorm together, and through building careers and families. Despite the distances and long intervals of being in touch, they have stood the test of time by responding and collaborating on this book with me.

I am also thankful to friends in Pakistan, London, The USA, and Canada who have been a continuous support in terms of helping for collaboration, data collection, proof-reading, and just being my support system in general during the journey of writing this book—Saira Shah, Tasneem Azim, Tazeen Kazi, Amina Khalid (Bima), Naureen Ahsan, Priyani Malik, and Nadia Bukhari.

Thank you is also due to my dedicated student research team: (1) Shahrukh Burki for her efforts in downloading relevant literature, helping in collecting participants for the practitioner survey (Chap. 6), and recording audio interviews with participants (Chap. 2); (2) Syed Asad Azeem Bukhari, Sadaf Qayum, and Soha Zubair for helping in organizing and presenting secondary data used in this book and tirelessly working on re-coding the Demographic Health Survey (DHS) files (Chap. 3); and (3) Habiba Taliya, Nimra Javed, Khadija Tanveer Chaudhry, Iqra Haroon Mazari, Syeda Fatima Raza Bokhari, and Bakhtyar Majeed for helping to enter data from SPSS to Excel files (Chap. 3).

Last but not least, thank you to the following women participants: (1) the four brave women who provided us with oral narrations for Chap. 2, (2) the woman microfinance borrower who allowed us to share her story for Chap. 4, and (3) the primary care practitioner participants from Chap. 6, who provided us with important information related to women's mental health challenges.

Contents

Contributors

Shaheda Anwar Department of Microbiology, Bangabandhu Sheikh Mujib Medical University, Dhaka, Bangladesh

Zamurrad Awan Department of Political Science, Forman Christian College University, Lahore, Pakistan

Fionnuala Gormley Global Market Risk Management Department, London, UK

Farooq Hasnat Department of Political Science, Forman Christian College University, Lahore, Pakistan

Sara Rizvi Jafree Department of Sociology, Forman Christian College University, Lahore, Pakistan

Tahira Jibeen Advance Health, Toronto, Canada

ClinicVillage Centre, Mississauga, Canada

Masha Asad Khan Applied Psychology Department, Kinnaird University, Lahore, Pakistan

Ainul Momina King Edward Medical University, Lahore, Pakistan

Bajiyanta Mukhopadhyay Cree Board of Health and Social Services, Waskaganish, Canada

Department of Family Medicine, McGill University, Montreal, Canada

Fareen Rahman Guy's and St Thomas' Hospital, London, UK

Deepti Sastry Independent Consultant, London, UK

Rubeena Zakar Institute of Social and Cultural Studies, University of the Punjab, Lahore, Pakistan

About the Editor

Dr. Sara Rizvi Jafree is an Assistant Professor in the Department of Sociology at Forman Christian College University (FCCU) in Lahore, Pakistan. She teaches courses related to Sociology of Gender, Health and Health Systems, Economic Sociology, and Sociology of Globalization. Having completed her BSc Honors in Economics from the London School of Economics and Political Science (LSE), Dr. Jafree pursued her MPhil and PhD in Sociology from University of the Punjab. An active researcher for funded projects in social welfare areas of microfinance and poverty alleviation, patient safety culture and workplace violence, and intergenerational learning for the elderly, she is also now working on her third book; her first book is titled *Women, Healthcare and Violence in Pakistan* (Oxford University Press, 2017). Dr. Jafree is part of the Lahore Biomedical Group and Special Needs Pakistan and is an Advisor to Rotary Club FCCU, all of which enable her to stay involved in community service and plan research objectives. Her current work is on digital health literacy interventions for special needs children and disadvantaged women seeking primary healthcare services, specifically in the context of infection prevention.

Chapter 1
Introduction

Sara Rizvi Jafree

When studying the sociology of societies, we must recognize that men and women of South Asia face different socio-environmental circumstances and life opportunities. So far health policy development efforts in South Asia have excluded cultural knowledge of women's unique circumstances. We rest the premise of this book on the fundamental understanding that South Asian social constructions of gender influence physical health, mental health, health adoption, and health recovery (Doyal 1995). Social and gender-based inequality in health stems from gender socialization patterns and gender differences in access to education and income. At a deeper level and for South Asia specifically, we must consider that basic social deprivations of family neglect, girl child undernutrition, and lack of physical activity also contribute to health inequalities in women from birth. Additionally, low self-esteem is absorbed by girls at a young age, due to low status allocation by significant others within the home, like parents and grandparents, making them less likely to adopt optimal health behaviors (Bhopal 2019). There is need for a systematic study of social barriers to better plan targeted interventions for health policies which are culturally cognizant and help to reform cultural factors which enable women to adopt health-seeking attitudes.

Health research has focused on planning health policy without keeping the socio-cultural factors and social systems influencing health access and health behavior in women at the forefront of policy development (Carrin and James 2005). Where health policy-makers are concerned with improving primary healthcare setup, referral systems, and health infrastructure, there has been less emphasis on understanding the social mechanisms which prevent women from reaching practitioners and health centers. It is also true that studies on South Asian women's health have targeted clinical evidence, with less attention on social and environmental factors driving health recovery and health outcomes. Holistic and comprehensive solutions to

S. R. Jafree (✉)
Department of Sociology, Forman Christian College University, Lahore, Pakistan

S. R. Jafree (ed.), *The Sociology of South Asian Women's Health*,
https://doi.org/10.1007/978-3-030-50204-1_1

health cannot be achieved without consideration of sociocultural and economic factors (Stotzer et al. 2013). Sociology being the systematic study of social systems, in this book we attempt to understand how the social structures of family, education, religion, economy, government, and media influence health behavior and health outcomes in women of South Asia. Additionally, we also aim to use the knowledge of social and environmental factors to recommend improved interventions and health policy for women of the region.

The South Asian region, more than any other part of the world, is driven by traditional and cultural forces which are possibly the most salient factors determining a woman's health awareness and her rights to adopt health behavior or pursue health recovery. Women of the region share a common culture and political history and there are benefits to understanding their problems collectively in order to design joint improvements in health policy for women. Any health system or substructure of society that does not consider human behavior and interaction is bound to remain inefficient and victim blaming. Since scholarship has concluded that health models must be preventive in their approach, there needs to be increased attention in South Asia on how women's lifestyle and behavior can be improved to aid preventive healthcare models (Watt 2002). If South Asia is to reduce its health costs and improve economic growth, health interventions for prevention must include an education and awareness-based approach which focuses on women's cultural circumstances and socially allocated positions in society.

With a population due to cross two billion people, South Asia is not only densely populated, but has forecasts for annual population growth rates expected at 1.2%. The people of the region are known to be rigidly patriarchal and conservative in their treatment and socialization of women (Bhopal 2019). It is well documented that the 920 million women living in the region face common and critical problems related to the feminization of poverty (Moghadam 2005) and the triple shift burden (Banu 2016). What is less known is that the women of the region are also plagued by the quadruple disease burden, with increasing rates of: communicable disease, noncommunicable diseases, violence and injuries, and maternal mortality (Cohen et al. 2017). South Asian women also face comparatively higher rates of multimorbidity compared to men and also show less gender gaps in life expectancy compared to women from the developed world. In addition, cultural customs such as girl child neglect, honor killing, revenge rape, and dowry victimization have exacerbated other gender-specific morbidity and mortality challenges. There is also concern that due to reporting barriers and punitive cultures we only know of the iceberg of illness and disease afflicting women of the region (Palermo et al. 2013).

The major emphasis for South Asian women's health by policy-makers has been on maternal mortality (Bhutta et al. 2004). Over a period of 25 years, maternal mortality rates in the region have declined successfully by 65%, as at 2013. Yet, there is little emphasis as to why health burdens for South Asian women related to communicable diseases, noncommunicable diseases, and accidents are on the rise (Engelgau et al. 2011; Solotaroff and Pande 2014; Zaidi et al. 2004). There is a simple answer for this. Maternal mortality has declined due to social support for improved fertility in women and all other health burdens have risen due to less cultural concern for holistic women's health quality of life and longevity. Different patriarchal forces determine health prioritization in women of South Asia, including family and in-laws, tribal leaders and feudal landlords, and male-dominated health policy-makers. There has also been little emphasis on researching how maternal health could be further improved if sociocultural reforms had been parallel to biomedical improvements and policy interventions. Decline in maternal mortality does not mean that statistics are favorable. There are still immense challenges to overcome due to social barriers to accessing pre- and postnatal healthcare, abortion care, assistance for birth spacing, and contraception (Akseer et al. 2017).

Though men are considered to have a lower life expectancy, it is women who have lower health quality during their life course (Selvaratnam 1988). In South Asia there is further complexity in comparing morbidity and illness due to underreportage in women. This underreportage has to a lot to do with honor codes and cultural values of keeping women's health a private domain. Historically, women with an illness or handicap have faced blame, stigma, and dishonor; and even in contemporary times fears of social shame create significant barriers in seeking healthcare and opting for health recovery (Rohwerder 2018; Stangl et al. 2019; Wynaden et al. 2005). Chronic diseases like cancers and diabetes, physical handicap, mental distress, and domestic and workplace violence are leading problems which cause women and girls to face great ostracization and stigma. In the event that an illness can be hidden and concealed, women and their families spend a lot of time and energy trying to hide the disease or handicap to avoid shame and dishonor (Banu 2016). This process of "passing" and pretending is also a cause of compounded health problems, lower health quality of life, and mental distress for women in the region.

Though there are benefits of grouping South Asian women together and designing health policy that would be relevant and beneficial to all, we must also consider the differences in geography, ethnicity, and class between women of the region (Bhutta et al. 2004). The question then for South Asia is how health equality can be guaranteed for all women? No doubt women from the upper classes and urban areas of South Asia have improved health access due to financial ease and geographical availability. Within class structures there are problems of the double standards in gendered perceptions for health access. Richer and urban women find it comparatively less difficult to gain social support for optimal and nontraditional health behavior and for not following the accepted social order of passivity and submissiveness. However, it is important to remember that South Asian women who are educated and from the upper classes may face considerable health barriers due to patriarchy and deprioritization of self (Fikree and Pasha 2004). This is because independent women from the region also perceive greater social acceptance and honor in accepting traditional roles of passivity in health-seeking behavior. Secondly, for many it is easier to accept historical patterns of role allocations and social expectations than to challenge social and family norms. Thirdly, even independent women may prefer to keep men as the central locus of their lives and accept patriarchal culture which determines health behavior in women. We must remember that as a collective body, women from South Asia perceive their social position and security to be attached with marriage and having a husband. More than God and religion or the self, it is the husband who is seen to as a demigod for salvation and safekeeping. The dominant joint family arrangement in South Asia further perpetuates control and submissiveness. This becomes a cause for deprioritization of self-health in women of all classes and also a cause for the relinquishing of health decision-making in the hands of husband's and in-laws.

Perhaps the greatest reason for South Asian society's deprioritization for women and girl's health is because of sustained and polemic son preference (Das Gupta et al. 2003). South Asia has high incidence of female feticide. There is little perceived functional utility of the girl child. Instead, with the dowry culture, daughters are considered to cost the family money and resources. To make matters worse, women of South Asia have become staunch proponents for the birth of a male child. This is because giving birth to a son still represents social status and acceptance for women and also provides them with perceived security for old age care and financial support. We may ask ourselves why South Asian women have not banded together to change perceptions and acceptance for the girl child? Why do mothers and sisters-in-law contribute to son preference? One of the reasons for this may be because mothers and sisters lose rank when their son or brother has a daughter and then grows to love the daughter (Sandhu 2014). Thus, not only do mothers and sisters have to share their son's and brother's time and affection, but the birth of nieces can also represent a challenge to the unquestioned authority and dominance over the kitchen, household finances, and management. Thus, not only son preference but lack of gender solidarity and the culture of South Asia women vying for control over men, to retain their security, further contribute to health negligence in women.

It is not expected that regressive norms and attitudes related to women's health behavior and health recovery will change very soon (Thornton and Fricke 1987). Having said this, there has to be a distinct way of planning health policy and care support for women in South Asia keeping sociocultural values at the forefront while retaining the positive aspects of local traditions and beliefs. Some examples of positive cultural customs include support through joint family arrangement, arranged marriage practices, and gerontocratic systems. All three have the advantage of retaining cultural customs and yet promoting health-seeking behavior. Arranged marriages and joint families can lead to collective family support for health-seeking behavior and health security of women, while gerontocratic culture can promote old age care within the family. Developing culturally relevant health policy with a social context for women in South Asia is necessary for acceptance and uptake of health. This is because Westernized health protocols for women's needs and Western medical aid and consultancy are not always well matched or accepted. There are also problems of fear and distrust that Western agents use healthcare investment as a means to control women's fertility and infectious disease (Kumar et al. 2016). This fear is supported by the heavy concentration of funding for maternal and child health, contraception, AIDS, and HIV.

Only an average of 60% of South Asian women have basic education and majority do not receive health literacy or education due to cultural barriers related to education for sexuality and reproduction (Unterhalter 2006). In many parts of the region, religious beliefs and the caste system prevent women from not just the uptake of family planning and reproductive health services, but also general health checkups and self-surveillance for disease (Sanneving et al. 2013). In these communities westernized educational models for health awareness or health literacy interventions are not effective (Engelgau et al. 2011), as they are considered alien to traditional models of passivity and self-neglect. There is need to introduce health literacy and health awareness in South Asia, but to develop a culturally sensitive model using secondary socializing agents like community notables, Jirga leaders, religious leaders, and media barons. It is therefore imperative for us that this book is a resource accessed not just by scholars and policy-makers for health, but a wider audience such as community notables and civilians.

Chapter two is an in-depth study of theories that explain South Asian women's health behavior. This chapter relies on using western theories and the available South Asian theories to explain health behavior of women. One of the reasons for South Asian theory lagging behind Western theory is because indigenous researchers have been reluctant to develop philosophical models and suffer prosecution from male-dominated community notables, religious leaders, and politicians. Multiple theories are used to explain the different health behaviors and choices of South Asian women, as the range of behavior patterns across regions and ethnicities is diverse and complex. Broad areas of influence covered in this chapter include: (i) culture and community, (ii) religion and the state, (iii) the individual woman herself, (iv) the capitalist economy, and (iv) transnational factors. This chapter is an important read for diverse populations such as students, practitioners, researchers, and policy-makers.

Chapter three presents oral narration by South Asian women with irreversible health conditions. There is no better way to understand the sociocultural factors influencing the health behavior, health recovery, and overall well-being of South Asian women with regard to their lived experiences of health than by hearing their voiced experiences. This chapter presents oral narrations of four women across South Asia with current health conditions of chronic nature or who have experienced major health setbacks in life. The women belong to diverse socioeconomic strata, which helps to put into context how social beliefs and attitudes transcend wealth and class. Two of the women participants face permanent health conditions from birth, paralysis and blindness; and the other two have developed health conditions after marriage, cancer and infertility. The findings reveal that the most complex and frustrating challenge for South Asian women has not been their health condition or lack of resources and health infrastructure, but the social and family support, public attitudes, and community acceptance which they have had to contend with through different stages of their health. Though the health experiences of all four women are different, they reveal the main challenges women face due to social customs, religious interpretations, and traditional values that are prevalent in South Asia.

Chapter four assesses South Asian women's decision-making for health. Though it is common to measure women's decision-making through variables, like choice in marriage, education, and employment, the variable of health decision-making has been less researched and emphasized. The complexity of health decision-making is that it is still considered a private domain. The strength of this chapter is that it uses recent secondary data from the Demographic Health Surveys of Bangladesh, India, and Pakistan to highlight predictors for health decision-making for women of reproductive age. This chapter discusses the salient cultural factors which influence or control health decision-making in women of South Asia: (i) gender gaps and family factor, (ii) health education and health behavior, (iii) nature of employment, (iv) violence and safety, and (v) quality of healthcare services and traditional healers. Necessary recommendations for health policy improvement for women of South Asia are recommended based on empirical evidence.

Chapter five investigates the role of poverty, health coverage, and credit opportunities in the lives of South Asian women, as important drivers for health access and relief. The chapter identifies the determinants of the feminization of poverty from a South Asian perspective which influences women's ability to access healthcare. Salient demographic and cultural areas include (i) family composition, (ii) control over resources, (iii) access to education and health, (iv) social protection inequality, and (v) labor market inequalities. Attempts at breaking the cycle of poverty are discussed in detail by describing the strengths and limitations of programs in Pakistan, Bangladesh, and India. The attempt in South Asia has been to compensate the lack of state provision for social and health security through microcredit opportunities. This chapter identifies critical problems that prevent the microfinance sector from facilitating emergence from poverty in women like informal sector employment, financial risks, and lack of or insufficient health insurance coverage. Secondary data has also been presented in this chapter along with a case-study from Pakistan on the lived health experiences of women microfinance borrowers.

Chapter six addresses the health challenges faced by refugee, displaced, and climate-affected women of South Asia. South Asia is one of the countries of the world suffering from substantial political mismanagement, ethnic conflict, natural disasters, and environmental degradation. Nearly 50 million refugees have crossed borders in South Asia since the colonial rule ended and are suffering from inadequate protection and services for health. Estimates from 2018 suggest that more than 10.3 million women of the region are currently suffering as a consequence of displacement caused by conflict or climate change. More women are suffering compared to men. The feminization of displacement has brought to attention that women compared to men during and after migration face considerable challenges in health experiences due to greater emotional and physical burdens and also due to greater vulnerabilities from violence and sexual abuse. Areas of disadvantages faced by displaced and migrant women are discussed in this chapter, in context to health challenges, including: (i) women-only households and lack of assets and information network, (ii) limited work opportunities and shortages of basic necessities, (iii) evacuation delays and life in temporary shelters, (iv) risk of violence, forced marriages and unplanned pregnancies, and (v) mental health and pressure of added care roles. Secondary data from UNHCR has also been used and a useful summary has been developed by the authors to classify the health impacts on women caused by environmental alterations due to displacement and climate change. The chapter recommends critical health reforms and extended health policy in the region for displaced women.

Chapter seven analyzes the social barriers to mental well-being for women of South Asia, an area which is grossly neglected. Health budgets in the region are negligible and rarely do any public or private sector health center have separate wards or practitioners for service delivery. This is despite the fact that women of South Asia are known to commonly face problems related to domestic violence, gender inequity, and sexual abuse, which places them at greater risk for mental health challenges. According to the literature the common and rising mental health challenges among South Asian women include: (i) post-traumatic stress disorder, (ii) dissociation disorders, (iii) conversion and depression, (iv) self-harm and suicide, and (v) eating disorders. This chapter investigates the social risk factors for mental distress in South Asian women, covering areas such as: status of the girl child, rites of passage, expectations of marriage, and nonconformity. The authors also examine the wider social and economic costs to society of neglecting women's mental health. Secondary data is used to present a comparative assessment of mental health challenges and incidence of women sufferers across South Asian states. The authors also present a case study containing a thematic analysis of the perceptions of women primary care providers regarding mental health of South Asian women. The chapter ends with recommendations for improved mental health policy for women of the region.

Chapter eight of the book addresses the sociology of political systems of South Asia and its influence on women's health behavior and health outcomes. Where the sociology of health is important for helping us consider that social factors determine health, such as gender, class, wealth, ethnicity, and literacy, it is the sociology of politics which helps us identify that public health policy is instrumental in closing the social gaps of health inequality. In this chapter the authors consider that in the capitalist democracies of the modern world, health is political because the planning and distribution of public health services is dependent on political intervention and also because some social groups have more access compared to others. The role of the state becomes more important especially in conservative and traditional milieus like South Asia where regressive cultural forces prevent women from maintaining optimal health or seeking health recovery. The chapter discusses key areas such as: (i) political representation; (ii) government budget for health; (iii) government licensing, regulation, and honesty; (iv) skewed population ratios; and (v) poverty and health financing. The authors also present a systematic recommendation for women's health policy reform at state level for South Asian countries.

The ninth and last chapter considers a rarely discussed area related to the culture and traditions of South Asia, which influence regulatory practices of the state. We argue that culture is responsible for sustaining regressive and inefficient regulatory policies in a nation and thus there needs to be a change in expectations and responsibility of state regulation for health. Types of regulation are discussed in-depth in order to map a proposal for an effective regulatory system for the health sectors of South Asia. The growth of commercialized providers and dual practice is driving much of the failure in health systems. More innovative approaches to regulation are needed in order to tackle traditions and legacy of lack of accountability and legitimized corruption in South Asia so that both public and private segments can start working effectively. The authors conclude about the utility of co-regulation in a decentralized manner, but with the state at the apex managing regulatory responsibility to the other actors in co-governance. The chapter's strength also lies in addressing the shortfalls of maternal health in South Asia by using secondary data from Demographic and Health Surveys. We propose recommendations for regulatory improvements by states in order to reduce the critical risk factors for maternal and child health.

References

Akseer, N., Kamali, M., Arifeen, S. E., Malik, A., Bhatti, Z., Thacker, N., et al. (2017). Progress in maternal and child health: How has South Asia fared? *BMJ, 357*, j1608.

Banu, A. (2016). *Human development, disparity and vulnerability: Women in South Asia*. Background paper for Human Development Report.

Bhopal, K. (2019). *Gender, 'race' and patriarchy: A study of South Asian women*. Routledge, Oxfordshire, UK.

Bhutta, Z. A., Gupta, I., de'Silva, H., Manandhar, D., Awasthi, S., Hossain, S. M., & Salam, M. (2004). Maternal and child health: Is South Asia ready for change? *BMJ, 328*(7443), 816–819.

Carrin, G., & James, C. (2005). Social health insurance: Key factors affecting the transition towards universal coverage. *International Social Security Review, 58*(1), 45–64.

Cohen, A. J., Brauer, M., Burnett, R., Anderson, H. R., Frostad, J., Estep, K., ... & Feigin, V. (2017). Estimates and 25-year trends of the global burden of disease attributable to ambient air pollution: an analysis of data from the Global Burden of Diseases Study 2015. The Lancet, *389*(10082), 1907–1918.

Das Gupta, M., Zhenghua, J., Bohua, L., Zhenming, X., Chung, W., & Hwa-Ok, B. (2003). Why is son preference so persistent in East and South Asia? A cross-country study of China, India and the Republic of Korea. *The Journal of Development Studies, 40*(2), 153–187.

Doyal, L. (1995). *What makes women sick: Gender and the political economy of health*. Macmillan International Higher Education, London, UK.

Engelgau, M., El-Saharty, S., Kudesia, P., Rajan, V., Rosenhouse, P., & Okamoto, K. (2011). *Capitalizing on the demographic transition: Tackling non communicable diseases in South Asia*. Washington, DC: World Bank.

Fikree, F. F., & Pasha, O. (2004). Role of gender in health disparity: The South Asian context. *BMJ, 328*(7443), 823–826.

Kumar, K., Greenfield, S., Raza, K., Gill, P., & Stack, R. (2016). Understanding adherence-related beliefs about medicine amongst patients of South Asian origin with diabetes and cardiovascular disease patients: A qualitative synthesis. *BMC Endocrine Disorders, 16*(1), 24.

Moghadam, V. M. (2005). *The 'feminization of poverty and women's human rights'*, SHS Papers in Women's Studies/Gender Research, (2).

Palermo, T., Bleck, J., & Peterman, A. (2013). Tip of the iceberg: Reporting and gender-based violence in developing countries. *American Journal of Epidemiology, 179*(5), 602–612.

Rohwerder, B. (2018). *Disability stigma in developing countries* (K4D Helpdesk Report). Brighton: Institute of Development Studies.

Sandhu, R. (2014). *Father attachment predicts adolescent girls' social and emotional development*. https://aura.antioch.edu/etds/93

Sanneving, L., Trygg, N., Saxena, D., Mavalankar, D., & Thomsen, S. (2013). Inequity in India: The case of maternal and reproductive health. *Global Health Action, 6*(1), 19145.

Selvaratnam, S. (1988). Population and status of women. *Asia-Pacific Population Journal, 3*(2), 3–28.
Solotaroff, J. L., & Pande, R. P. (2014). *Violence against women and girls: Lessons from South Asia*. Washington, DC: World Bank.
Stangl, A. L., Earnshaw, V. A., Logie, C. H., van Brakel, W., Simbayi, L. C., Barré, I., & Dovidio, J. F. (2019). The health stigma and discrimination framework: A global, crosscutting framework to inform research, intervention development, and policy on health-related stigmas. *BMC Medicine, 17*(1), 31.
Stotzer, R. L., Silverschanz, P., & Wilson, A. (2013). Gender identity and social services: Barriers to care. *Journal of Social Service Research, 39*(1), 63–77.
Thornton, A., & Fricke, T. E. (1987). *Social change and the family: Comparative perspectives from the West, China, and South Asia.* Paper presented at the Sociological forum.
Unterhalter, E. (2006). *Measuring gender inequality in education in South Asia*. Citeseer.
Watt, R. G. (2002). Emerging theories into the social determinants of health: Implications for oral health promotion. *Community Dentistry Oral Epidemiology, 30*(4), 241–247.
Wynaden, D., Chapman, R., Orb, A., McGowan, S., Zeeman, Z., & Yeak, S. (2005). Factors that influence Asian communities' access to mental health care. *International Journal of Mental Health Nursing, 14*(2), 88–95.
Zaidi, A. K., Awasthi, S., & deSilva, H. J. (2004). Burden of infectious diseases in South Asia. *BMJ, 328*(7443), 811–815.

Chapter 2
South Asian Women's Health Behavior: Theoretical Explanations

Sara Rizvi Jafree and Deepti Sastry

2.1 Introduction

The sociology of health developed as a specialized subject after the Second World War (Horobin 1985). The political and economic turmoil across the world necessitated the theorizing of health solutions based on a rational social science. The need was that populations should remain healthy through preventive healthcare or recover as soon as possible in order to return to the workforce through curative healthcare. The Chicago School was a forerunner for academic pursuits in sociology of health research, whereas the US and European economies were where the hospital-based policy improvements were initiated. The 1970s and 1990s saw revivals in the sociology of health, the former due to the growth in critical sociology (Twaddle 1982) and the latter due to the post Fordism consumer culture (Annandale and Field 2001).

According to many researchers the sociology of health has received the least attention and development (Halsey 2004). This may be because of the perceived social urgency to concentrate on specializations like the sociology of development, political sociology, and social stratification. Consequently, the sociology of women's health and the health of South Asian women has received even less attention. Though limited theories are available by South Asian scholars, it is still imperative to consider theoretical explanations or constructs from the developed world which might help us to explain the health behavior of South Asian women (Prochaska et al. 2002). One of the reasons for South Asian scholarship lagging behind may be because indigenous researchers have been reluctant to develop philosophical models and suffer prosecution or ostracization from male-dominated community

S. R. Jafree
Department of Sociology, Forman Christian College University, Lahore, Pakistan

D. Sastry (✉)
Independent Consultant, London, UK

S. R. Jafree (ed.), *The Sociology of South Asian Women's Health*,
https://doi.org/10.1007/978-3-030-50204-1_2

notables, religious leaders, and politicians. In this way, we must rely on using western theories, already established and published, which can be referenced with ease, but manipulated slightly to relate to the South Asian context. Since one theory cannot explain the different behaviors and choices of South Asian women, as the range of behavior patterns across regions and ethnicities is diverse and complex, we will consider broad areas of influence in this chapter, including: culture and community, religion and the state, the individual woman, new age health problems, and, finally, transnational factors.

There is also the matter of defining a healthy South Asian woman through different life stages in a subjective and fluid postmodern world. Essential definitions of healthy woman include the availability of social factors such as: nurturing parents, adequate food and nutrition, clean water, shelter and seasonal clothing, and support from socializing agents with regard to health awareness and health decision-making rights. However, never-ending debates between liberals and conservatives regarding the preference of western-centric health models versus traditional health models, and family imposed decision-making versus personal choice, have prevented indigenous researchers from investigating South Asian woman's health. Though similarities between women of the world and South Asia can be generalized, there are salient differences in the social and cultural predictors of health for South Asian women, compared to women from other regions of the world. What is unique about South Asia is that it has a distinctive history and culture, which have together influenced the people's beliefs, practices, and social interaction. The culture of patriarchy, the interpretation of religious beliefs, and the feudal and gerontocratic nature of families have placed women's health and well-being at the back seat of academia, legislation, and policy-making.

A chapter that attempts to present sociological theories explaining the health behavior of South Asian women rests on what the empirical evidence tells us. The theories discussed in this chapter will address why South Asian women suffer from the following critical problems: (i) female feticide and girl child mortality; (ii) malnutrition and food insecurity; (iii) neonatal and maternal health problems; (iv) mental health problems; (v) osteoporosis and arthritis; (vi) infectious and communicable diseases, specifically respiratory and gastroenteritis, and HIV and AIDS; (vii) chronic illnesses like heart disease, breast and lung cancer, and diabetes; and (vii) lack of timely health seeking behavior and inefficient healthcare services. Figure 2.1 is a summary flowchart which presents the broad social factors and the related theories under each factor, influencing South Asian women's health.

2.2 Culture and Community

South Asia's oldest religious belief systems which have combined to influence the health behavior of women in the region include Hinduism, Buddhism, and Islam. The Hindu ideology depicted through the laws of Manu prohibited the education and social mobility of women. Women were unable to access healthcare unless it

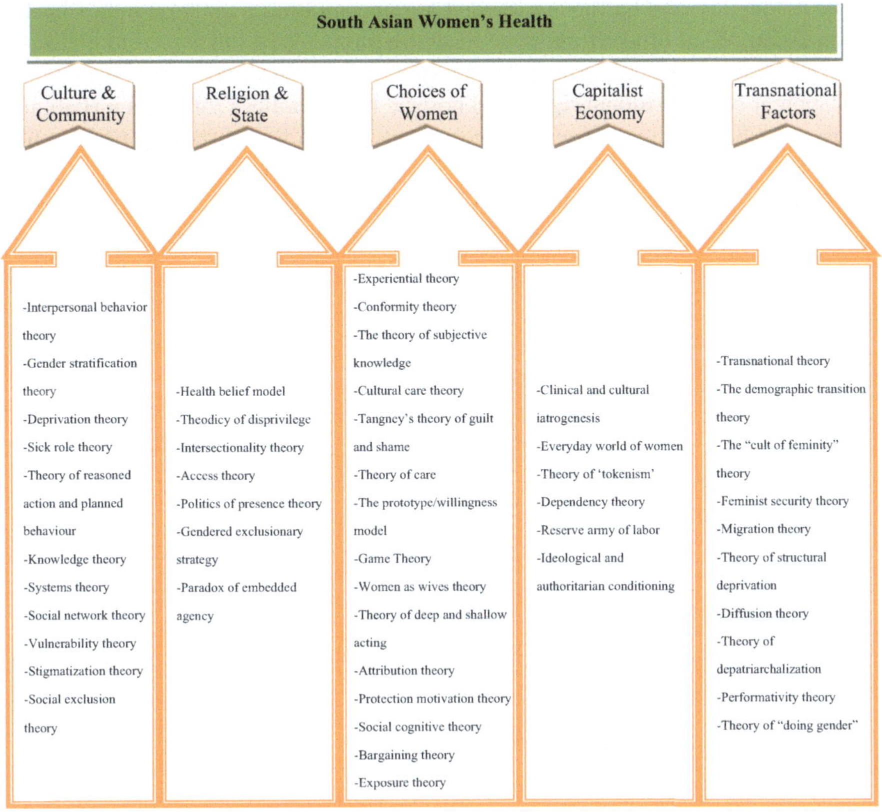

Fig. 2.1 Flowchart describing the relationship between theory and social factors influencing the health behavior and outcomes of South Asian women

was by local women healers (Niaz 2003). Buddhist ideologies taught men to distance themselves from women in order to attain salvation. Women's health was not a priority for Buddhist missionaries and women were not allowed to be cared for in Buddhist temples (Tsomo 2012). Muslim invaders brought regressive pagan Arab beliefs against women to the subcontinent and contributed to the misogynistic beliefs and practices of existing communities. Legitimization by untrained Muslim religious leaders further condoned violence and abuse against women in South Asia. Women were segregated and excluded from decision-making. Their primary roles were considered as reproductive agents. Barren women were set aside and replaced, through remarriages, whereas women who suffered complications and died in childbirth were remembered as noble women who died fulfilling their family and religious roles. Ultimately, the two dominant religious ideologies of South Asia, Hinduism and Islam, have tended to exclude women in political participation and governance decision-making, which has had an effect on health policy-making and public health provision for women (Haque 2013).

The colonial period has been recorded as concentrating mainly on men's health (I. Sen 2010). What little efforts were made for women's health served to highlight the benevolence of the colonizers and the need for women nurses, as opposed to the development of professional rights and holistic health polices for women (Pati and Harrison 2008). During the freedom movement women were used as a tool for liberation and as partners of men. However, post the colonial period women were once again relegated to secondary citizenship status, with constitutional rights and policy development for women, including health policy, a forgotten goal. To make matters more complicated, the current health service protocols for women and research on maternal health in South Asia have basically been inherited by the West (Maddison 2013). This has created great resistance to what is seen as Westernized health practices and services for women, contributing to the social barriers related to access and permission for healthcare.

The theory of interpersonal behavior claims that behavior is influenced by factors of intent, habit, and facilitating conditions (Triandis 1977). Intent and habit are strongly influenced by the conditioning and learning from primary and secondary socializing agents, such as parents, family, teachers, peers, work colleagues, and the community. Unconsciously, women follow a sequence of health behaviors that they have habitually seen their family and community follow. South Asian societies are known to deprioritize the girl child from nutrition and healthcare leading to greater mortality, morbidity, malnourishment, and adverse sex ratios (B. Agarwal 1994). *The theory of gender stratification* helps us understand why women and the girl child are given less preference for basic human rights such as: food, healthcare, and education (Blumberg 1984). It seems that the main reason might be that all these basic rights cost money, whereas majority South Asian women either do not earn an income or are informally employed and underpaid. Women of the region are also deprived of other sources of income for health financing through wealth and property ownership as they inherit less. Overall, South Asian families are known to invest in the health of male members of the family more, as men are considered more important for family succession, inheritance maintenance, and old age support of parents and other relatives.

We may use the *deprivation theory* to argue that like the working classes, women are an inferior class, who are not supported in attaining skills, education, and employability (Raju 1991). As a result, South Asian society has justified regressive practices against women, which have adverse and multiple health consequences, such as: (i) child marriage, (ii) intimate partner violence and domestic violence, (iii) neglect of symptomatic signs of ill health, (iv) preference of unlicensed practitioners for maternal health and child delivery, and (v) rejection of western biomedicine, vaccinations, and immunizations. It is also true that many South Asian families believe that keeping women within the home, not letting them go for health checkups outside the home, and not letting them visit male practitioners and hospital settings will protect their women and their families from loss of honor (Balayla 2011).

The *sick role theory* suggests that once a person has been categorized as sick, they receive family, community, and employer benefits and support for recovery (McKinlay 1972). However, the theory neglects to consider that all women cannot so easily adorn the "sick role," as they are not socially supported in this. South Asian women are considered the sole domestic providers and categorization of legitimate illness by a medical practitioner would mean the need for substitution of their domestic labor. It is because of this lack of willingness of society to substitute asymmetrical domestic work that women have difficulties in accessing healthcare providers and in turn getting assigned the "sick role." In cases where they are permitted a "sick role," they still do not get leave from domestic work and have to continue with their roles despite ill health and fear of compromised recovery.

The theory of reasoned action and planned behavior helps to highlight the role of beliefs and social norms in women's intentions for seeking healthcare (Fishbein and Ajzen 1975). As South Asian belief systems are dominated by forceful and rigid patriarchal ideologies, the women of the region develop more powerful intents to control their own health according to the customary and prevalent social order. This can be seen in the belief of many South Asian women that immunization and vaccination cannot benefit their children (Ahmadian and Samah 2013). Also, South Asia is still a region where women prefer to deliver their child at home, with unskilled unlicensed attendants instead of in an institution, despite the risks (Jafree et al. 2018). However, as women move into urbanized zones, receive education, and learn from media and peers about biomedical healthcare and the importance of scientific evidence, they may start to opt for safer health practices such as institutional deliveries or the utilization of skilled attendants in the homes and community.

Majority of South Asian women suffer from compartmentalized knowledge or limited access to information regarding health, nutrition, and well-being. *Knowledge theory* has described that access to knowledge is the main influencing factor in shaping beliefs and meanings. As women are trained through the hidden curriculum, within the home and at primary school, about cultural norms related to their health, by their family, community, and kin, they become ideologically conditioned to pursue traditional health practices (Miranda et al. 2006; Shipton and Goheen 1992). Knowledge about health recovery and health risks is essential for women to adopt health seeking behavior. The ability to have health knowledge and be able to act upon it, however, is dependent on many things such as: rural-urban belonging, local development and educational access, family literacy, media exposure, and adherence to regressive values and the traditional order. Research from South Asia shows that when women have more awareness and access for early breast examinations, there is higher detection at earlier stages of cancer and improved survival rates (Hossain et al. 2014).

Systems theory helps to describe the relationship between South Asian woman and filial piety, in relation to her health choices and her role as an informal healthcare provider in the family (R. Gupta and Pillai 2000). Decisions for South Asian women's health is strongly influenced by her elders and their respective understanding pertaining to women's health. The systems approach also helps us to recognize that the health of South Asian women will only undergo systematic changes over time if the environment, culture, and social relationships change. South Asian traditions of filial piety are not something that necessarily need to be abandoned. But we must recognize that conditioning through filial piety can have both positive and negative effects, negative if the family traditions are negligent of women's health and positive if the traditions are supportive of women's health.

Social network theory suggests that community and kinship are important in keeping South Asian women connected to their traditions and identity (Krause et al. 2007). The possibility of being excluded from the network and losing ties means the loss of family and community. South Asian women need to be a part of strong social networks for encashment in life events like poverty, emergencies, religious and cultural festivals, and marriages and funerals. Women who do not want to be excluded from the community network will emulate the patterns of health behavior that exist in their network in order to retain social relationships and kinship solidarity (Granovetter 1983; Smith-Lovin and McPherson 1993). They will rarely attempt to break valuable community networks in order to retain or regain health, and this includes traditional preferences for home delivery, rejecting consultancies from male medical practitioners, and avoiding invasive tests like mammography and pap smears. Conversely, if women are lucky to have a social network which promotes healthcare and health access they can benefit from reduced stress, guidance during emergency and acute health problems, early identification of disease, and ongoing sharing of health information (R. Gupta and Pillai 2000).

Fineman's theory of vulnerability suggests that disadvantaged and marginalized women do not have the opportunities to make decisions in their own interests and thus government social welfare tools must ensure that such women gain health services (Kohn 2014). However, since South Asia is not known as a prototypical region for state-initiated social welfare policies, the accountability falls on family members. Women's dependent status on their families due to economic poverty and gender segregation powerfully influences their household inequality and ability to gain health services (Cunha and Garrafa 2016). According to researchers in South Asia women who do not have decision-making rights in the household are unable to seek trained practitioner assistance for maternal and child health and overall family health (Bloom et al. 2001; Fikree and Pasha 2004; Hou and Ma 2011). Even working women in South Asia, with independent incomes, commonly permit their male relatives and in-laws to make decisions regarding their life choices and health behavior. Researchers have found that financially autonomous women assume decision-making rights for their child's schooling, but that they forgo rights for decisions related to self-health (Hou and Ma 2011). This could be because the women of South Asia fear the informal sanctions associated with independent decision-making.

With regard to health, perhaps more than in any other region of the world, women of South Asia are fearful of the social stigma associated with disease and illness. Chronic illnesses, like cancer, are diseases that women can barely talk about, let alone seek treatment for. Many women, unaccounted for, prefer to die rather than seek treatment for cancer. This is mostly explained by *stigmatization theory* (Goffman 1997) and the concepts of "covering," "passing," and "withdrawal," each of which explains how women choose to engage in assuming normalcy, hiding the disease, and avoiding social interaction, respectively. South Asian women are known to suffer extreme stigma and shame when diagnosed with cancer, especially breast and ovarian cancer, as it can compromise fertility and reproduction, and for many women unexplained death is a better option than seeking treatment and disclosing illness (Bedi and Devins 2016; Hann et al. 2018). Additionally, the cost of treatment for chronic diseases and cancer, travel distance for healthcare, the time and assistance needed from working male members of the family, makes both access difficult and the seeking of healthcare less of a preference for women.

Social exclusion theory has been popularly used in South Asian research to explain the problems marginalized populations like women, elderly, and the transgender communities suffer from in society (Johnston 2009). Social exclusion leads to lack of access to education, employment, and healthcare. In addition, social exclusion can become a cause for loss of dignity and self-esteem, which leads to considerable mental health problems in women and other marginalized populations. The theory also highlights how the family and community blacklist women from health seeking behavior; this may be due to one or all reasons such as honor, veiling, and unwillingness to spend money on women. Unfortunately, social exclusion can not only prevent women from seeking access to healthcare at primary level, but create permanent and compounding problems of health at the tertiary level and adds to the burden of chronic disease. An example is women who are unable to seek the proper gynecological and pelvic examinations for cysts and fibroids can suffer subsequent health problems like permanent infertility and undiagnosed uterine cancer.

2.3 Religion and State

The health belief model helps to explain why some women believe health is a matter related to religious piety (Kirscht et al. 1966). Primary agents in South Asia, like parents, grandparents, aunts, and uncles, through the socialization process have instilled values in the youth that women only suffer health problems and infertility when they are not pious. Knowledge of religious traditions, steadfastness in prayers, and observance of religious vows (*mannat*), pilgrimage to the graves of local saints, and the use of amulets (*taweez*) are considered the overarching domain and distinction of women in many South Asian families. The health belief model describes four components that influence health behavior, including: (i) severity of illness, (ii) susceptibility to illness, (iii) benefits of prevention, and (iv) barriers to taking health assistance. Taking the case of early detection of breast cancer, South Asian women's decision to have an ultrasound and mammography is influenced by their belief and attitudes regarding exposing the breast and letting it be handled by practitioners. This prevents them from gaining benefits of early detection and chance for cure. Knowledge of family history of cancer can only benefit a woman when she believes that she can change her lifestyle and eating habits and adopt preventive and early diagnosis measures. In many cases South Asian women's beliefs may restrict them to herbal and traditional (*hakeem*) medicine and prayer as a treatment for breast lumps.

Weber suggests the *theodicy of disprivilege* to describe how women use participation in religious rituals and prayer as a means to compensate for their powerlessness. In the quest for worldly status through religious piety many South Asian women may neglect primary visits to the practitioner and early detection of illness (Turner 2011). In addition, the revival of religious extremism, politicization of religious ideologies, and ethnic conflict, in the last few decades, have contributed to both the negligence of health policies related to women and also to extreme oppression and violence against them (Zaman 1999).

Intersectionality theory proposes that there are interlocking systems in a society which can disadvantage women (Hancock 2016). Systems can play a crucial role in simultaneously working to oppress women and prevent them from adopting healthy lifestyles and seeking health assistance. These multiple sources of explosive disadvantage include culture, ethnicity, class, language, education, employment, ability to spend their own money, decision-making rights, mobility, religion, governance, and laws. The South Asian woman that is more oppressed socially and politically, in her region of origin or as a migrant, will have fewer options for health and well-being (Lockhart and Danis 2010). The inadequate legal constitutions across regions of South Asia and the lack of legal enforcement of bills, if they exist, has placed South Asian women at the mercy of traditional customs.[1] The enforcement and superior power of Jirga laws and traditional laws in many areas places women at grave risk of mortality and morbidity through practices like honor killing, wata satta,[2] revenge rape, and dowry and bride price (Iqbal 2007).

Ribot and Peluso have talked about *access theory*, which is the ability of people to benefit through access to property, people, and institutions (Ribot and Peluso 2003). There are two aspects of access we are concerned with: firstly, whether women have access to land, wealth, and health facilities and health practitioners and, secondly, if they do not, whether it is the state's responsibility to ensure that women have these rights as citizens of the state. The theory forces us to consider state negligence when women cannot access other civilian rights, such as: (i) rights to report crime and violence and (ii) rights to report deprivation of basic necessities related to health and well-being, including education and employment, public transport, tube wells, groundwater, electricity, and water pumps (Dubash 2002; In Ribot and Peluso). Cultural barriers to ownership of land, property, and other resources, like cars and businesses by daughters, wives, mothers, and sisters, are a complex problem in South Asia. Refugees, migrants, and IDPs can suffer from complete lack of access to health facilities and services (Carballo and Nerukar 2001). Research from the region shows that though some South Asian women can gain access to microfinance loans, they do not always benefit from improved health quality of life due to lack of health insurance and

---

[1] Traditional practices which place women at greater health risks include: child marriage, polygamy, dowry provision, high fertility and low birth spacing, and domestic violence.

[2] Watta Satta is a type of forced marriage through exchange, where a brother and sister from one household are married to another brother and sister from a second household. This arrangement can become a source of extreme reciprocal violence against the women involved.

savings, excessive work burden, and pressure to repay loans at high installment rates (Jafree and Ahmed 2013).

The governments of South Asia are perhaps the most important drivers for social change though policy mobilization. A state-led policy for compulsory screening of domestic violence victims can reduce domestic abuse and change cultures. *The politics of presence theory* stresses that when women are excluded from parliament, governance, and policy-making, it creates systematic gender inequality across the structures and laws of the country (Phillips 1995). Women of South Asia are rarely found in governance positions, making their contribution in health policies and planning for women a serious concern in the region. The public healthcare systems have grave shortfalls in relation to health access and insurance coverage. When available and accessible the public health services are known to have serious problems of low budget allocations, corrupt practices, inefficient services, and shortages in staffing and resources. Private health services, including consultancy and surgery, are difficult to access due to cost, transport problems, and time (Fikree and Pasha 2004). Another concern is that health services in South Asia have concentrated on fertility health and not on other health problems of significance to women. One such example is the lack of screening for domestic violence in public and private hospitals of South Asia, which has directly supported the culture of violence and lack of reporting by victims (Jafree 2018).

Anne Witz further describes through her theory of *gendered exclusionary strategy* that women are excluded in the professions of medicine and medical administration (Witz and Savage 1991). While professions like nursing, paramedics, and midwifery are reserved for women, these vocations do not have direct influence on health policies. Poststructuralist feminist theory from the region has described the dependency of women and the community on the traditional birth attendant (TBA) for preservation of traditional customs (V. Agarwal 2017; A. Sen 2012). In most regions the TBA is more powerful than the medical practitioner. The South Asian woman trusts that the TBA will secure her health through maintenance of a traditional diet and vaginal delivery, as opposed to imposing practices that are against culture, religion, and traditions. It is because of this that there is no clear dichotomy between biomedical healthcare and traditional healthcare for the women of South Asia. *The paradox of embedded agency* helps explain how powerful and rigid social structures, such as the public and private health centers, can be influenced by individuals, medical practitioners, and traditional healers (Keshet 2013). In smaller health centers of South Asian communities, the lady doctors and traditional birth attendants have partnered to produce a hybrid professional identity of biomedicine and traditional healthcare. Even larger hospitals of South Asia are known to provide complementary and alternative medicine as a means to facilitate and appease traditional families and provide accepted forms of health assistance for women (Roy et al. 2015). The embedded nature of women as agents of change and innovation has played a role in sustaining traditions and also transforming health centers from conventional western models.

2.4 Choices of the South Asian Woman

Experiential theory addresses that it is not just the cognitive process that influences learning and behavior, but that there is a significant role played by social experiences and emotions (Sladek et al. 2010). Emotions and experiences are possibly the most important factor determining the health behavior in South Asian women. The people of the region are ruled by emotions derived from ties of blood and kinship, and primarily it is the South Asian woman who is responsible for negotiating relationships much more than their male counterparts. Women are expected to maintain peace and harmony within the family and in the community. It is this emotion that forces the South Asian woman to voluntarily shoulder a much higher burden of unpaid care work.

In the new millennium it is still the South Asian woman who takes responsibility for duties that perhaps more liberal and western women do not take any more.[3] Most of this unpaid care work takes long hours and receives little recognition or appreciation. This leaves us with the question of how much time women realistically have for health seeking behavior. Research suggests that women in the region have less time to visit practitioners or health centers and make changes regarding healthy choices in diet and lifestyle (Basu 1992). The traditional and cultural expectations of ceaseless unpaid care work from South Asian women are understood to make them more vulnerable to poverty and unemployment. However, what is less researched is that it also places them at constant risk of disease and illness, as they are unable to prioritize preventive health behavior and health seeking behavior. Why do women place themselves at such risk despite growing awareness about the importance of self-health? *Conformity theory* suggests that women recognize that if they break customs and traditions, they run the risk of losing their social status and also compromising the reputation of their family and children. The theory can be used to explain how South Asian women conform and contain themselves from seeking healthy lifestyles and health services in order to fit in and be appreciated as the sacrificing and ideal South Asian woman, who are upholding legacies of their predecessors (Bernheim 1994).

The theory of subjective knowledge (Flynn and Goldsmith 1999) helps to explain that illiterate, semiliterate, and untrained women become confident in their subjective opinions for health practices when judgments and decisions by traditional attendants coincide with traditional practices of health (Aertsens et al. 2011). The choice that South Asian women have taken is to reject modern biomedical solutions and hospital deliveries, even when healthcare services are available in urban slums. *Leininger's theory of cultural care* further helps to explain why South Asian women

[3] Some of the items on the list of unpaid care work include: (i) looking after the home (cooking, cleaning, laundry, ironing, grocery shopping, and supervision of servants); (ii) taking care of the children, house, in-laws, parents and siblings, and sick family members; (iii) regular visitation and assistance to relatives and neighbors (cooking, babysitting); and (iv) taking part in religious and cultural events being celebrated or observed in the community or among relatives.

choose traditional healers over medical practitioners, as they feel that their religious, philosophical, and traditional customs for health and recovery are observed by the traditional healers (Leininger 1995).

Tangney's theory of guilt and shame suggests that women can feel guilt in some cultures due to the strain of having to maintain family traditions and kinship bonds (Tangney 1998). Any deviant behavior and violation of traditional social norms means the shaming of not just the woman, but also the family. Many South Asian women assume a persona of seclusion and passivity, in order to avoid all chances of assuming responsibility and guilt during different life circumstances. As times have changed and women are required to be more mobile, educated, and employed, the risks to them becoming a source of shame for their family can multiply. This is perhaps why significant working women of South Asia do not feel pride and gain self-esteem in sharing the household financial burden, but instead feel shame and guilt in neglecting the home during paid employment outside the home (Samman et al. 2016). This shame can become a source of paralysis in adopting assertive behavior for health and instead become a source for retaining traditional attitudes toward healthcare (T. J. Ferguson et al. 2000).

Carol Gilligan's theory of care confirms that a dominant ethic of care in women shapes their identity and behaviors across all spheres of their life (Tronto 1987). The explosive combination of care provision and the need to provide emotional labor means that South Asian women do not prioritize health seeking behavior. South Asian women are socialized to be more emotional and nurturing, and this can also instill in them more sentiments of guilt and shame. In addition, their primary role as care providers means that they only have time to prioritize the health of their family members and not themselves. In other words, prioritizing their own health needs would mean loss of their identity and status in their household and family. This is why many women prefer not to seek cancer treatment and chemotherapy, as the disease protocol requires both time and money, and it robs them from their primary roles as care providers to others (Taber et al. 2015).

The prototype/willingness model suggests that women may be more willing to take greater health risks (Gerrard et al. 2008). This willingness may be prompted by social events, social images, and social expectations. South Asian women who choose to give birth at home may be aware of the risk to themselves and their child, but are willing to take the risk in order to avoid social censure and gain social honor. A normal delivery at home without the cost, time, and exposure to outsiders would gain women more status within their family and in-laws. Similarly, women who have seen their elders become addicts to intoxicants like heroin and tobacco still may pursue unhealthy habits in order to cope and survive difficult social circumstances of poverty, uncertainty, and unemployment.

Marriage is an important life event for South Asian women, if not the most important factor in determining her status and inclusion in society. *Game theory* as described by Sen helps us to understand how the South Asian woman perceives herself to have a weaker bargaining position in marriage (A. K. Sen 1987). Women from the region desire to get married and remain married as this is associated with their personal status and family honor. Marriage takes precedence over women's personal choice and satisfaction in marriage. According to *Greene's theory of "women as wives"* a strong ideology exists representing marriage as the most important female role (Greer and Inglis 1971). The ideal wife and mother are expected to suffer and sacrifice for their children and if the children turn out bad they are expected to "take the blame." Not only are women as daughters and wives neglected in terms of health by society, but as mothers they individually make a choice to place themselves last on the priority list for health awareness and health financing. Duncombe and Marsden in their *theory of deep and shallow acting* argue that women pass through two stages, first during courtship or the early days of marriage and the next as time passes during their marriage (Duncombe and Marsden 1993). In the initial stages of their relationship women experience the "deep act," where they avoid doubts about their spouse, and in the later stages they experience the "shallow act," where they pretend that their relationship is satisfactory. South Asian women are extremely dependent on projecting the mirage of a perfect marriage in order to preserve their reputation and social honor. They also are eager to gain the approval of their husbands in order to secure financial support and the well-being of their children. This causes women to accept the rulings and decisions of husband and in-laws and to even normalize discriminatory behavior such as the absence of permission and financial support for health access.

Attribution theory describes how individuals explain the causes of their behavior, either through the circumstances they are in, external attribution, or through personal characteristics, internal attribution (Kelley 1967). In many instances women are barred from gaining health services due to external barriers of structural access and family permission. Women's health behavior can be improved when they recognize the power of internal attribution. The improvement of maternal and child health services by the state and community is not something individual women can change so easily. However, women who recognize the benefits of prenatal and postnatal medical care will assume individual responsibility through practitioner and institutional checkups. *Protection motivation theory* further describes responses to a health threat based on, first, a woman's appraisal of the threat and the severity of illness and, second, on the ability to cope with the treatment (Rogers 1975). This may be one of the reasons why cancer and rheumatoid arthritis is detected very late in women of South Asia (Dos Santos Silva et al. 2003). Low awareness makes women ignore the initial symptoms and fear of social shame and lack of finances makes them reluctant to seek treatment.

Social cognitive theory helps to explain how South Asian women execute health behavior based on their self-efficacy (Bandura and Adams 1977). Self-efficacy is the belief in one's ability to do something and is developed from social interactions and experiences. The theory suggests that health behavior is influenced by the knowledge that women acquire about the consequences of their actions. Women who continue to eat oil-based food and do not adopt exercise regimes, despite being diagnosed with high blood pressure and high cholesterol, do not believe they are capable of changing their diet and lifestyle (Lawton et al. 2008). The belief that their previous matriarchal generations also ate the same traditional food and led the same sedentary lifestyle contributes to their inability to take control and change their lives toward health management.

Liberalist and neoliberal feminist ideologies have described the modern and urban-based South Asian woman as a new age woman who is seeking autonomy and self-fulfillment (H. Gupta 2016; Harvey 2007). In order to gain a professional identity and maintain it, she is fast learning the benefits of: (i) maintaining a healthy lifestyle, (ii) early screening for disease, and (iii) not compromising on relationships that inflict physical and mental abuse. According to *bargaining theory*, women with better education, employment, and social status are able to make better choices for healthcare for themselves and their children (Rose 1994). In addition *exposure theory* (Hornik 2002) suggests that a woman with more exposure to the world through literacy, media, and mobility can make better health decisions for herself, in terms of researching health problems, travelling to different practitioners, seeking specialized assistance, reading prescriptions and ingredients of medicine, and following practitioner's instructions for home care, nutritional and lifestyle changes, and follow-ups.

2.5 The Capitalist Economy

One of the results of the development of the contemporary biomedical model has been the dependency on scientific explanations and male-dominated explanations of health and disease. From these explanations stem the belief of mind-body dualism and the treatment of the body as a complicated machine. The result was that women's bodies were placed under the control of the powerful and autonomous male medical practitioner. Health issues like menstruation and pregnancy began to be treated as a sickness, while headaches and hysteria were seen as problems related to the uterus and ovaries (Ehrenreich and English 1978). *Illich's theory of clinical and cultural iatrogenesis* suggests that the medical profession and the cultural dependency on the medical model can actually do more harm than good for a woman's health (Milligan 1998). Research suggests that women who do not need caesarian sections and hysterectomies are made to believe that they do by powerful surgeons and medical practitioners, thus leading to unnecessary surgeries and compounded health problems.

The liberal feminists have always contended that women with comparative economic advantages, in terms of wealth and occupational status, have better health standards compared to women who have neither. There is a problem however of women's economic subordination in South Asia, first, due to segregation and, second, due to inferior work opportunities. Dorothy Smith (1987) discussed the *everyday world* of a woman (Harding 2009), which is a gendered space depending on the woman's region and community of origin (Fernandez and Campero 2017). The theory suggests that a woman's private space is influenced by political and historical realities that surround her locality. In most South Asian communities, a woman's domestic space is where she has relative control and honor. Contrarily, she faces exclusion, discomfort, and even violence in public and work spaces. This forces a woman to remain in her comfort zone within the domestic sphere, which means she is less eager and willing to not only seek health access outside the home, participate in the formal workforce, and take active part in mobilizing health improvements for women from political epicenters. Working women in South Asia, compared to the nonworking women, also deliver low birth weight children due to lack of nutrition and pre- and postnatal healthcare and also the absence or inadequacy of maternal and employment benefits (Jafree et al. 2018).

Kanter's theory of "tokenism" at male-dominated workplaces suggests that women are only employed to superficially show that the institution is gender neutral (Kanter 1977). The problem with tokenism is that no concrete steps are taken by the organization to promote policies for protection and promotion of women, including health insurance and medical benefits for working mothers (Zimmer 1988). Elderly women especially in South Asia who have never had an income or belonged to the formal sector of the economy suffer from health deprivation due to lack of health insurance and savings. Many prefer not to become a financial burden for their relatives or ask for assistance in being taken for medical checkups and tests, as it would mean male family members taking leave from work and possibly losing daily wages. In this way they may choose not to seek health solutions or seek health solutions from cheaper and local neighborhood healers, quack doctors, and unlicensed health providers. In all, the influence of capitalism compels society and state to force women to become economically productive while still shouldering her traditional domestic duties single-handedly (Baksh-Soodeen and Harcourt 2015). There is little doubt that the accepted culture of patriarchy for many South Asian women leaves their health needs conditions in the hands of men, their fathers, brothers, husbands, and sons. In addition, the workplace is also dominated by the male employer and male heads of organization. Ultimately, health policy development by the capitalist economy is usually directed to the well-being, protection, and development of men, not women.

Women in the underdeveloped regions of South Asia are now facing multiple burdens, including having to participate in the workforce for paid income, for example, working in local factories. Despite the presence of local basic health units (BHUs) and maternal health clinics, women are so burdened by domestic and formal or informal work outside the home that they are unable to seek health services. Furthermore, the lack of infrastructure in underdeveloped and rural regions of South Asia means that women are susceptible to more health problems due to lack of support systems in the home, such as: electricity, water pipes, gas heating and cooking stoves, clean water for drinking, gutter and drainage system, washing machine, and dish washers (Ramey 2009). The less the technology available in the home, the less time women have for health seeking behavior and adoption of a healthy lifestyle. A woman who spends most of her day carrying water to the home, and collecting wood for cooking fire, will have less time to spend on cooking something healthy for herself or her family. Thus, if women have time and energy to cook only one meal a day, they will prioritize family preference for the meal over their own health needs. In addition, with less household income, cheaper and unhealthy food is known to be a more practical option for women responsible for home management (Afridi et al. 2018; Hu 2003).

Marxist feminists have used *dependency theory* to show how globalization has negatively impacted women from developing regions due to the gender-based inequalities practiced by transnational companies and capitalist firms (Singh 2007). Women are employed in the lowest paying jobs with inferior or no employment benefits. Margret Benston and Lesley Doyal explain how the capitalist system benefits from the free labor of women in the homes (Benston 1989). Women who are in paid work are usually found in unskilled jobs with unsafe work environments, including: domestic labor, factory production, agricultural labor, and secretarial posts. The capitalist and free market economy thrives on free domestic labor that women provide and the cheap labor they contribute to in the workforce (Sarker 2006). The capitalist model has benefited from the patriarchal culture by neglecting to develop state and organizational policies for women's employee benefits and safety, including healthcare, and in many cases by neglecting to provide health coverage for wives and other dependents.

Doyal's theory of the *reserve army of labor* clarifies how women's primary role is reproduction and that the medical and pharmaceutical industry supports capitalism in focusing predominantly on reproductive and fertility health of women (Doyal 1995). The capitalist industry requires women to reproduce the next generation of workers and benefits from the free labor that women provide at home, so that their men can come to work happy and healthy. According to Doyal the cumulative efforts of domestic work, reproduction, and paid work production in the economy have a deleterious effect on women's health. Despite this burdensome role and the consequent susceptibility to ill health, women do not seek healthcare for themselves due to theoretical explanations of *ideological and authoritarian conditioning*. According to David Cooper and Diane Feeley, women are ideologically taught their subservient role by their primary and secondary socializing agents, in the homes and at schools, and they thus learn to remain submissive and nonassertive in health seeking as this is not their ideal role in a capitalist society (Lapidus 1978).

2.6 Transnational Factors

Transnational theory emphasizes that the identities and behavior of women are also influenced by social activities that take place across political borders, geographical spaces, and diverse cultures (Messias 2002). Politics, international relations, foreign policy, and global media are all combining to have an effect on every aspect of women's social existence, most especially health and well-being. It is not only migrants and travelers who are influenced by global discourses and actions for women's health, but media has closed the gap between ignorance and awareness. The *demographic transition theory* has predicted that fertility rates will decline as healthcare improves and urbanization spreads (D. Kirk 1996). The pressures of poverty and modernization have pulled women into the workforce in South Asia, contributing to a decline in fertility rates, though average family sizes are still far greater compared to other regions of the world (Offenhauer and Buchalter 2005). In South Asian countries sons are considered an asset, not just in terms of helping hands for household income, but also due to social status and family honor. Fertility is high because of low preference for family planning desire for larger families, but for women also because having more children is a personal choice as it grants them higher honor and status in the household and community. Higher fertility for mothers is a well-documented risk for maternal mortality, and it also compromises the health quality of life for women and their aging process (Stokoe 1991). Women who have more children and suffer more miscarriages and abortions suffer from greater rates of osteoporosis, gynecological complications, weakness and fatigue, nutritional deficiencies, anemia, and hypertension.

Marjorie Ferguson while describing the *cult of femininity* (M. Ferguson 1983) suggests that women are directing by media, literature, and magazines to value themselves according to their beauty, cooking skills, management of home, and number of children born. Media in the contemporary world plays a significant role in developing the conscious identity and behavior patterns of women. The simulations of health management and the recovery process for a sick person is not something that is represented by the media as a valued feature of the "ideal" South Asian woman. It is because of this that many South Asian women avoid seeking healthcare services, in order to retain the social image of their selflessness and perfection. This may also be why they turn to local quacks and religious healers as primary contacts and quick solutions for health relief, often with dire consequences to their continued health and mortality (Wasti et al. 2015).

South Asia is home to extreme conflict and terrorism, and according to arguments by international conflict feminists like Vasuki Nesiah, it is the women who suffer the most insecurity and violence (Nesiah 2006). Gendered insecurity has profoundly negative physical and psychological health impacts on women, through which feminist struggles for equalities post the colonial era have been critically undermined (Jafree 2018; Simister and Makowiec 2008). *Feminist security theory* highlights how women living in or affected by conflict are deprived in terms of: (i) basic resources, like food, water, housing, and welfare, and (ii) having to live in perpetual fear and insecurity (Sjoberg and Via 2010). Fear cripples women and girls as they are unable to access healthcare and citizenship rights. There are also crippling fears that women will be used as tools for revenge and plunder. According to some South Asian women (Zaman 1999), it is preferable to commit suicide after rape or kidnapping, as women become social misfits and are severely ostracized by the community after their abuse due to cultures of victim blaming in South Asia. Ironically, it is the victimized woman, who is given the responsibility to become an agent of peace in regions of conflict and violence (J. Kirk 2004). Thus, as South Asia women are given additional burdens of peace and recovery in conflict regions of South Asia, their own health can become less of a priority for them due to added burdens of being nominated as peace and recovery agents.

South Asian populations have been plagued with civil unrest, regional instability, political turmoil, poverty and ethnic exclusion, and even genocide. Millions of families are suffering from displacement, refugee status, and voluntary or involuntary migration. Women refugees and migrants are understood to suffer greater health risks from displacement, compared to men, as they (i) are less likely to have savings accounts or be able to get paid employment and (ii) are known to be used for trafficking, sexual slavery, and as objects for barter and revenge during wars. In addition, due to the missing women and the demographic shortfall of women in some parts of South Asia, there is an illegal market for the supply of women. Forced migration and kidnappings have caused numerous health problems for women including physical trauma and permanent psychological problems (Kapila 2013). Though kidnapped women who are forced into marriage or prostitution are not migrants, most of them are not living in their native community anymore. Thus, *migration theory* alerts us that such women, stripped of their surroundings, community, and family, may suffer extreme cases of discrimination and oppression (Boyd and Grieco 2003). In addition, the *theory of structural deprivation* is useful in explaining how migrants, displaced women, and women refugees are not being provided with state protection, legal accountability, and state healthcare (Gurin 1985).

According to modern-day South Asian theorists, South Asian women have become more cognizant of their health due to improved access to higher education, economic participation, professional specialization, exposure to media, and changes in ideologies (Jeffery and Basu 1996). *Diffusion theory* (Ilie et al. 2005) helps to explain how South Asian women through modernization and global convergence are adapting to health seeking behaviors by opting for marriage only after securing permanent employment with maternal benefits. Such women also choose to give birth at the hospital, practice birth spacing, plan smaller families, and visit trained practitioners for pre- and postnatal checkups to secure their health in the long run.

In the *theory of depatriarchalization* feminist theorists have shed light on how democratization has motivating gender equality and awareness of rights for citizenship (Matos and Paradis 2014). Women's development movements have made efforts to deconstruct traditional constructions of health behavior post colonization and to allow women to have health awareness and rights (Mohanty 2005). The process of decolonizing feminism in Pakistan has become the project of some women rights groups, who are gradually moving toward efforts for women's holistic health. However, the role of male policy drivers, politicians, media, religious leaders, and community notables is critically important in driving change toward optimal and positive health seeking behavior and opportunities for the women of South Asia.

According to *performativity theory* a woman's gender identity is socially constructed through a series of ongoing performances (Butler 2006). Based on their regional differences South Asian women construct their own knowledge about health behavior derived from discourses of health, well-being, and quality of life. The more modern, urbanized, and educated the South Asian woman, the better health knowledge she will have due to access to advanced local and global health discourses. Undoubtedly, the South Asian woman is faced with a duality in identities as she may try to adapt to some protocols for health and yet try to retain her traditional and cultural identity. This can be seen in an example where a woman would be willing to take consultancy from a male medical practitioner, but choose to take delivery assistance from a "lady doctor," even if the latter was less skilled and experienced.

South Asian women are regularly producing new subjectivities concerning health and well-being. Some of them have taken strides to abandon traditionally regressive and religious understandings of health in order to align themselves with Western classifications of good health. Participating in sports and eating nutritious food are changes in health behavior that women are bringing into the lives of their daughters, despite it not being a reality during their own growth years (Babakus and Thompson 2012). Other women have adopted yoga and classical dancing with the dual aim of reviving culture and also for maintenance of health (Newcombe 2017). It would not be entirely wrong to say that the more urbanized and modern the South Asian woman, the less social backlash and stigmatization she may face for *doing gender* and adopting independent and progressive health seeking behavior (Senarath and Gunawardena 2009).

2.7 Conclusion

Theoretical frameworks that explore gender have largely focused on the lived realities of Western white women, followed by some exploration of the gendered lives of black women, while less emphasis has been placed on brown woman. Though research on South Asian women is growing, researchers are still reluctant to widen the scope of their analyses. Reasons include frequently changing daily realities for South Asian women, the rapid nature of change in the postmodern era, and the enormous differences in ethnicities, culture, and religious beliefs in the region. There have been substantial changes in gender theories of health, from structural theories to actor theories and, finally, to postmodern theories. However, what all of them have in common is an assertion that society, structures, and the environment play a significant role in influencing the health choices and challenges faced by South Asian women.

By the middle of the twentieth century women had become part of the workforce, even in the traditional and segregated spaces of South Asia. If in the past women's health was primarily important for childbearing and enduring of domestic burdens, it took on new dimensions of importance as women started assuming additional roles to uphold the national economy. Ultimately, empowering all the genders with health is an economic and social necessity to ensure both increased productivity, the maintenance of the capitalist economy, and to ensure that the quality of life indicators for women's health is improving across the world.

Low quality of life as it relates to health for women in South Asia and high mortality rates have been theoretically explained by their cultural relegation to secondary citizenship both within the household and in the community. The association between health, life opportunities, and resource deprivation has been explored, including integral and current areas of relevance, such as: water shortages, climate change, regional conflict and displacement, educational systems, financial autonomy, media choices, and role burden. The difficulty in health access due to lack of patronage by religious leaders and the state has been highlighted; however, significant barriers for South Asian women happen to be individual choices by women themselves. Ideological conditioning, early socialization, and the self-fulfillment of regressive social expectations have deprioritized health. The limitations of colonialism, capitalism, and the Western biomedical model have shown that women have inherited problems, which have become difficult to tackle in the face of new age and transnational issues which places greater economic and social pressure on women, leaving little time and energy for health seeking behavior.

There are different types of South Asian women to consider when associating theoretical frameworks for understanding health behavior, the traditionally poor, the modern elite, and the middle classes. The first is unable to adopt healthy lifestyles due to poverty, illiteracy, lack of choice, and awareness; the second is adopting health seeking behaviors, as she is educated, aware, and part of a modern social network which supports her choices; and the third consists of many categories of middle-class women who lie somewhere in between and are making choices daily between neglect, traditional health choices, and modern biomedical models. The theories discussed in this chapter confirm that gender allocated norms for health access and healthcare are not so easily changed or improved in South Asian societies. Behavior patterns are curtailed, regulated, and controlled by culture, religion, family, state structures, and personal choices. Overall, the social construction of ill health for women, both physical and mental, are still very negative in South Asia, making it difficult for women to actively pursue or invest in health recovery, even when there is access for themselves and the girl child.

In this way, we have much to discuss and look forward to in the rest of this book. There may very well be a critical problem of an illness iceberg in South Asia, where women's health problems are neither reported, assessed, or planned for. Without cultural and social reform women of the region will never feel encouraged or comfortable to adopt health seeking behavior. Finally, the theories examined in this chapter point to the critical problem of the continuum of care for South Asian women. No doubt there is a structural problem of lack of record keeping and referral for specialized consultancy in the public health sector, but there is also the issue of women not being able to seek continuous care or follow-up for a timely healthcare regime. This is not just due to an inefficient healthcare setup, lack of time and energy, and the absence of finances, but because of lack of social acceptance and support for continuous and consistent health prioritization in women over their life span.

References

Aertsens, J., Mondelaers, K., Verbeke, W., Buysse, J., & Van Huylenbroeck, G. (2011). The influence of subjective and objective knowledge on attitude, motivations and consumption of organic food. *British Food Journal, 113*(11), 1353–1378.

Afridi, F., Dinkelman, T., & Mahajan, K. (2018). Why are fewer married women joining the work force in rural India? A decomposition analysis over two decades. *Journal of Population Economics, 31*(3), 783–818.

Agarwal, B. (1994). Gender and command over property: A critical gap in economic analysis and policy in South Asia. *World Development, 22*(10), 1455–1478.
Agarwal, V. (2017). Breaking boundaries: Complementary and alternative medicine provider framing of preventive care. *Qualitative Health Research, 27*(13), 2019–2029.
Ahmadian, M., & Samah, A. A. (2013). Application of health behavior theories to breast cancer screening among Asian women. *Asian Pacific Journal of Cancer Prevention, 14*(7), 4005–4013.
Annandale, E., & Field, D. (2001). Medical sociology in Great Britain. In *The Blackwell Companion to medical sociology* (pp. 246–262). Londres: Blackwell Publishers.
Babakus, W. S., & Thompson, J. L. (2012). Physical activity among South Asian women: A systematic, mixed-methods review. *International Journal of Behavioral Nutrition Physical Activity, 9*(1), 150.
Baksh-Soodeen, R., & Harcourt, W. (2015). *The Oxford handbook of transnational feminist movements*. Oxford: Oxford Handbooks.
Balayla, J. (2011). Male physicians treating female patients: Issues, controversies and gynecology. *McGill Journal of Medicine: MJM, 13*(1), 72.
Bandura, A., & Adams, N. E. (1977). Analysis of self-efficacy theory of behavioral change. *Cognitive Therapy Research, 1*(4), 287–310.
Basu, A. M. (1992). *Culture, the status of women, and demographic behaviour: Illustrated with the case of India*. Oxford: Clarendon Press.
Bedi, M., & Devins, G. M. (2016). Cultural considerations for South Asian women with breast cancer. *Journal of Cancer Survivorship, 10*(1), 31–50.
Benston, M. (1989). The political economy of women's liberation. *Monthly Review, 41*(7), 31–44.
Bernheim, B. D. (1994). A theory of conformity. *Journal of Political Economy, 102*(5), 841–877.
Bloom, S. S., Wypij, D., & Gupta, M. D. (2001). Dimensions of women's autonomy and the influence on maternal health care utilization in a north Indian city. *Demography, 38*(1), 67–78.
Blumberg, R. L. (1984). A general theory of gender stratification. *Sociological Theory*, 23–101.
Boyd, M., & Grieco, E. (2003). Women and migration: Incorporating gender into international migration theory. *Migration Information Source, 1*(35), 28.
Butler, J. (2006). Performative acts and gender constitution: An essay in phenomenology and feminist theory. In *The RoutledgeFalmer reader in gender & education* (pp. 73–83). New York: Routledge.
Carballo, M., & Nerukar, A. (2001). Migration, refugees, and health risks. *Emerging Infectious Diseases, 7*(3 Suppl), 556.
Cunha, T., & Garrafa, V. (2016). Vulnerability: A key principle for global bioethics? *Cambridge Quarterly of Healthcare Ethics, 25*(2), 197–208.
Dos Santos Silva, I., Mangtani, P., De Stavola, B., Bell, J., Quinn, M., & Mayer, D. (2003). Survival from breast cancer among South Asian and non-South Asian women resident in South East England. *British Journal of Cancer, 89*(3), 508.
Doyal, L. (1995). *What makes women sick: Gender and the political economy of health*. Macmillan International Higher Education.
Dubash, N. K. (2002). Tubewell capitalism: Groundwater development and agrarian change in Gujarat. New Delhi: Oxford University Press.
Duncombe, J., & Marsden, D. (1993). Love and intimacy: The gender division of emotion and emotion work' a neglected aspect of sociological discussion of heterosexual relationships. *Journal of Sociology, 27*(2), 221–241.
Ehrenreich, B., & English, D. (1978). The sick women of the upper classes. *The Captive Imagination: A Casebook on "The Yellow Wallpaper". 96.*
Ferguson, M. (1983). *Forever feminine: Women's magazines and the cult of femininity.* Ashgate Pub Co.
Ferguson, T. J., Eyre, H. L., & Ashbaker, M. (2000). Unwanted identities: A key variable in shame–anger links and gender differences in shame. *Sex Roles, 42*(3–4), 133–157.
Fernandez, R. M., & Campero, S. (2017). Gender sorting and the glass ceiling in high-tech firms. *ILR Review, 70*(1), 73–104.

Fikree, F. F., & Pasha, O. (2004). Role of gender in health disparity: The South Asian context. *BMJ, 328*(7443), 823–826.
Fishbein, M., & Ajzen, I. (1975). *Intention and behavior: An introduction to theory and research*. Reading: Addison-Wesley.
Flynn, L. R., & Goldsmith, R. E. (1999). A short, reliable measure of subjective knowledge. *Journal of Business Research, 46*(1), 57–66.
Gerrard, M., Gibbons, F. X., Houlihan, A. E., Stock, M. L., & Pomery, E. A. (2008). A dual-process approach to health risk decision making: The prototype willingness model. *Developmental Review, 28*(1), 29–61.
Goffman, E. (1997). Selections from stigma. *The Disability Studies Reader, 203*, 215.
Granovetter, M. (1983). The strength of weak ties: A network theory revisited. *Sociological Theory, 1*, 201–233.
Greer, G., & Inglis, A. (1971). *The female eunuch*. London: Paladin.
Gupta, H. (2016). Taking action: The desiring subjects of neoliberal feminism in India. *Journal of International Women's Studies, 17*(1), 152–168.
Gupta, R., & Pillai, V. K. (2000). Caregiver burden in South Asian families: A systems theory perspective. *Journal of Ethnic Cultural Diversity in Social Work, 9*(1–2), 41–53.
Gurin, P. (1985). Women's gender consciousness. *Public Opinion Quarterly, 49*(2), 143–163.
Halsey, A. H. (2004). *A history of sociology in Britain: science, literature, and society*. Oxford: Oxford University Press.
Hancock, A.-M. (2016). *Intersectionality: An intellectual history*. Oxford: Oxford University Press.
Hann, K. E., Ali, N., Gessler, S., Fraser, L. S. M., Side, L., Waller, J., et al. (2018). Attitudes towards a programme of risk assessment and stratified management for ovarian cancer: A focus group study of UK South Asians' perspectives. *BMJ Open, 8*(7), e021782.
Haque, S. T. M. (2013). Theories of governance: South Asian perspective. *Public Organization Review, 13*(4), 365–379.
Harding, S. (2009). Standpoint theories: Productively controversial. *Hypatia, 24*(4), 192–200.
Harvey, D. (2007). *A brief history of neoliberalism*. Cary: Oxford University Press.
Hornik, R. C. (2002). Exposure: Theory and evidence about all the ways it matters. *Social Marketing Quarterly, 8*(3), 31–37.
Horobin, G. (1985). Medical sociology in Britain: True confessions of an empiricist. *Sociology of health illness, 7*(1), 94–107.
Hossain, M. S., Ferdous, S., & Karim-Kos, H. E. (2014). Breast cancer in South Asia: A Bangladeshi perspective. *Cancer Epidemiology, 38*(5), 465–470.
Hou, X., & Ma, N. (2011). *Empowering women: The effect of women's decision-making power on reproductive health services uptake: Evidence from Pakistan*. Washington, DC: The World Bank.
Hu, F. B. (2003). Overweight and obesity in women: Health risks and consequences. *Journal of women's health, 12*(2), 163–172.
Ilie, V., Van Slyke, C., Green, G., & Lou, H. (2005). Gender differences in perceptions and use of communication technologies: A diffusion of innovation approach. *Information Resources Management Journal, 18*(3), 13–31.
Iqbal, N. (2007). Legal pluralism in Pakistan and its implications on women's rights. *Scratching the Surface: Democracy, Traditions, Gender, 101*.
Jafree, S. R. (2018). *Women, healthcare, and violence in Pakistan*. Karachi: Oxford University Press.
Jafree, S. R., & Ahmed, K. (2013). *Women microfinance users and their association with improvement in quality of life: Evidence from Pakistan*.
Jafree, S. R., Zakar, R., Mustafa, M., & Fischer, F. (2018). Mothers employed in paid work and their predictors for home delivery in Pakistan. *BMC Pregnancy Childbirth, 18*(1), 316.
Jeffery, R., & Basu, A. M. (1996). *Girls schooling womens autonomy and fertility change in South Asia*.
Johnston, H. B. (2009). Addressing social exclusion: Analyses from South Asia and southern Africa. *Journal of health, population, nutrition, 27*(4), 423.

Kanter, R. (1977). Men and women of the corporation. *Publishers of New York*, P245–P266.
Kapila, K. (2013). … In South Asia. *HAU: Journal of Ethnographic Theory, 3*(2), 299–304.
Kelley, H. H. (1967). *Attribution theory in social psychology.* Paper presented at the Nebraska symposium on motivation.
Keshet, Y. (2013). Dual embedded agency: Physicians implement integrative medicine in health-care organizations. *Health, 17*(6), 605–621.
Kirk, D. (1996). Demographic transition theory. *Population Studies, 50*(3), 361–387.
Kirk, J. (2004). Promoting a gender-just peace: The roles of women teachers in peacebuilding and reconstruction. *Gender Development, 12*(3), 50–59.
Kirscht, J. P., Haefner, D. P., Kegeles, S. S., & Rosenstock, I. M. (1966). A national study of health beliefs. *Journal of Health Human Behavior, 7*, 248–254.
Kohn, N. A. (2014). Vulnerability theory and the role of government. ***Yale Journal** of Law & **Feminism**, 26*(1).
Krause, J., Croft, D. P., & James, R. (2007). Social network theory in the behavioural sciences: Potential applications. *Behavioral Ecology Sociobiology, 62*(1), 15–27.
Lapidus, G. W. (1978). *Women in Soviet society: Equality, development, and social change.* Berkeley: University of California Press.
Lawton, J., Ahmad, N., Hanna, L., Douglas, M., Bains, H., & Hallowell, N. (2008). 'We should change ourselves, but we can't': Accounts of food and eating practices amongst British Pakistanis and Indians with type 2 diabetes. *Ethnicity health, 13*(4), 305–319.
Leininger, M. (1995). Overview of Leininger's culture care theory. In M. Leininger (Ed.), *Transcultural nursing concepts, theories, research & practices* (College custom series) (2nd ed., pp. 93–112). New York: McGraw-Hill.
Lockhart, L. L., & Danis, F. S. (2010). *Domestic violence: Intersectionality and culturally competent practice*. New York: Columbia University Press.
Maddison, A. (2013). *Class structure and economic growth: India and Pakistan since the Moghuls.* Routledge.
Matos, M., & Paradis, C. G. (2014). Challenges for the Depatriarchalization of the Brazilian State. *Cadernos Pagu, 43*, 57–118.
McKinlay, J. B. (1972). The sick role—Illness and pregnancy. *Social Science Medicine, 6*(5), 561–572.
Messias, D. K. H. (2002). Transnational health resources, practices, and perspectives: Brazilian immigrant women's narratives. *Journal of immigrant health, 4*(4), 183–200.
Milligan, F. (1998). The iatrogenic epidemic. *Nursing Standard, 13*(2), 46.
Miranda, A. O., Bilot, J. M., Peluso, P. R., Berman, K., & Van Meek, L. G. (2006). Latino families: The relevance of the connection among acculturation, family dynamics, and health for family counseling research and practice. *The Family Journal, 14*(3), 268–273.
Mohanty, C. T. (2005). *Feminism without borders: Decolonizing theory, practicing solidarity.* Zubaan.
Nesiah, V. (2006). Truth commissions and gender: Principles, policies, and procedures. *International Center for Transitional Justice, 18*, 7–8.
Newcombe, S. (2017). The revival of yoga in contemporary India. *Oxford Research Encyclopedia of Religion.*
Niaz, U. (2003). Violence against women in South Asian countries. *Archives of Women's Mental Health, 6*(3), 173–184.
Offenhauer, P., & Buchalter, A. R. (2005). *Women in Islamic societies: A selected review of social scientific literature.*
Pati, B., & Harrison, M. (2008). *The social history of health and medicine in colonial India.* London: Routledge.
Phillips, A. (1995). *The politics of presence*. Oxford: Clarendon Press.
Prochaska, J. O., Redding, C. A., Evers, K. E., Glanz, K., Lewis, F., & Rimer, B. (2002). *The transtheoretical model stages of change*. In *Health behavior and health education: Theory, research, and practice* (pp. 60–84). San Francisco: Jossey-Bass.

Raju, S. (1991). Gender and deprivation: A theme revisited with a geographical perspective. *Economic Political Weekly, 26*, 2827–2839.
Ramey, V. A. (2009). Time spent in home production in the twentieth-century United States: new estimates from old data. *The Journal of Economic History, 69*, 1–47.
Ribot, J. C., & Peluso, N. L. (2003). A theory of access. *Rural Sociology, 68*(2), 153–181.
Rogers, R. W. (1975). A protection motivation theory of fear appeals and attitude change1. *The Journal of Psychology, 91*(1), 93–114.
Rose, C. M. (1994). Bargaining and gender. *Harvard Journal of Law & Public Policy, 18*, 547.
Roy, V., Gupta, M., & Ghosh, R. K. (2015). Perception, attitude and usage of complementary and alternative medicine among doctors and patients in a tertiary care hospital in India. *Indian journal of pharmacology, 47*(2), 137.
Samman, E., Presler-Marshall, E., Jones, N., Bhatkal, T., Melamed, C., Stavropoulou, M., & Wallace, J. (2016). *Women's work: Mothers, children and the global childcare crisis*. London: Overseas Development Institute.
Sarker, D. (2006). Development theory and gendered approach to development: Some theoretical issues in the Third World's perspective.
Sen, A. K. (1987). Gender and cooperative conflicts (Helsinki: World Institute for Development Economics Research, Working Paper No. 18).
Sen, I. (2010). Memsahibs and health in colonial medical writings, c. 1840 to c. 1930. *South Asia Research, 30*(3), 253–274.
Sen, A. (2012). Martial tales, right-wing Hindu women, and "history telling" in the Bombay slums. *South Asian Feminisms: Contemporary Interventions*, 75–94.
Senarath, U., & Gunawardena, N. S. (2009). Women's autonomy in decision making for health care in South Asia. *Asia Pacific Journal of Public Health, 21*(2), 137–143.
Shipton, P., & Goheen, M. (1992). Introduction. Understanding African land-holding: Power, wealth, and meaning. *Africa, 62*(3), 307–325.
Simister, J., & Makowiec, J. (2008). Domestic violence in India: Effects of education. *Indian Journal of Gender Studies, 15*(3), 507–518.
Singh, S. (2007). Deconstructing 'gender and development' for 'identities of women'. *International Journal of Social Welfare, 16*(2), 100–109.
Sjoberg, L., & Via, S. (2010). Conclusion: The interrelationship between gender, war, and militarism. In *Gender, war, militarism: Feminist perspectives* (pp. 231–239). Santa Barbara: ABC-CLIO.
Sladek, R. M., Bond, M. J., & Phillips, P. A. (2010). Age and gender differences in preferences for rational and experiential thinking. *Personality Individual Differences, 49*(8), 907–911.
Smith, D. E. (1987). The everyday world as problematic: A feminist sociology. University of Toronto Press.
Smith-Lovin, L., & McPherson, J. M. (1993). You are who you know: A network approach to gender. *Theory on gender/feminism on theory*, 223–251.
Stokoe, U. (1991). Determinants of maternal mortality in the developing world. *Australian New Zealand journal of obstetrics gynaecology, 31*(1), 8–16.
Taber, J. M., Leyva, B., & Persoskie, A. (2015). Why do people avoid medical care? A qualitative study using national data. *Journal of general internal medicine, 30*(3), 290–297.
Tangney, J. P. (1998). How does guilt differ from shame? In *Guilt and children* (pp. 1–17). Amsterdam: Elsevier.
Triandis, H. C. (1977). *Interpersonal behavior*. Monterey: Brooks/Cole Publishing Company.
Tronto, J. C. (1987). Beyond gender difference to a theory of care. *Signs: Journal of Women in Culture Society, 12*(4), 644–663.
Tsomo, K. L. (2012). *Buddhist women and social justice: Ideals, challenges, and achievements*. SUNY Press.
Turner, B. S. (2011). Max Weber and the spirit of resentment: The Nietzsche legacy. *Journal of Classical Sociology, 11*(1), 75–92.

Twaddle, A. C. (1982). From medical sociology to the sociology of health: Some changing concerns in the sociological study of sickness and treatment. In *Sociology: The state of the Art* (pp. 324–358). London: Sage.

Wasti, H., Kanchan, T., & Acharya, J. (2015). Faith healers, myths and deaths. *Medico-Legal Journal, 83*(3), 136–138.

Witz, A., & Savage, M. (1991). The gender of organizations. *The Sociological Review, 39*(1_suppl), 3–62.

Zaman, H. (1999). *Violence against women in Bangladesh: Issues and responses.* Paper presented at the Women's Studies International Forum.

Zimmer, L. (1988). Tokenism and women in the workplace: The limits of gender-neutral theory. *Social Problems, 35*(1), 64–77.

Chapter 3
Oral Narrations of Social Rejection Suffered by South Asian Women with Irreversible Health Conditions

Sara Rizvi Jafree and Fareen Rahman

3.1 Introduction

There is no better way to understand the sociocultural factors influencing the health behavior, health recovery, and overall well-being of South Asian women with regard to their lived experiences of health than by hearing their voiced experiences. It is evident that the most complex and frustrating challenge for South Asian women is not their health condition or lack of resources and health infrastructure, but the social and family support, public attitudes, and community acceptance which they have to contend with through different stages in their lives. Though the health experiences of all four women are different, they reveal the main challenges women face due to social customs, religious interpretations, and traditional values that are prevalent in South Asia.

The primary data for this chapter will be based on qualitative research, which provides rich data about lived experiences and practices (Polkinghorne 2005). Qualitative interviews are especially useful for gender-based research in areas of health, well-being, and social integration, which needs deeper exploration and insights (Mauthner and Doucet 2003). All women who narrated their experiences in this chapter are suffering from chronic health conditions or have experienced major health setbacks in life. The women belong to diverse socioeconomic strata, which helps to put into context how social beliefs and attitudes transcend wealth and class. Two face permanent health conditions from birth, paralysis and blindness, whereas the other two have developed health conditions after marriage, cancer and infertility. Audio recordings were used to assist in transcription of the interviews with the

S. R. Jafree
Department of Sociology, Forman Christian College University, Lahore, Pakistan

F. Rahman (✉)
Guy's and St Thomas' Hospital, London, UK

S. R. Jafree (ed.), *The Sociology of South Asian Women's Health*,
https://doi.org/10.1007/978-3-030-50204-1_3

permission of participants. All women were informed of the research objectives and were assured they could leave the interview at any point during the proceedings. Anonymity and confidentiality were guaranteed, and for the sake of preservation, names and regions have not been shared. In addition, some demographic details have been altered in order to further preserve the anonymity of women participants.

Ethics approval for this study was sought from The Institutional Review Board, Forman Christian College University. Two participants were recruited through health support groups on Facebook, and two were purposively sampled through purposive networking (Elgesem 2015). Internet-mediated research is recognized as a valid and credible means of collecting primary data (Hewson 2003). Informed consent for participation in the study was taken through an online form or an email confirmation, as was convenient for participants (Speer and Stokoe 2014). There is great advantage that Internet research allows for researchers who need to sample people from locations they cannot access (Andrews et al. 2007). The interviews were held by phone, as the authors did not belong to the same city as participants, and travelling for interviews was not a possibility for authors. Women participants were requested to provide a suitable time for the interview, when they were in a private settings and based on their convenience and ease. Additionally, many participants prefer to talk to interviewers without face to face interaction and through telephone, as they are able to select their time of interviews and also ensure that no one is overhearing their conversations (Tausig and Freeman 1988). Permission for audio recordings of telephonic interviews was also taken and these recordings have only be used for analysis of data. All audio recordings are stored with the first author and will not be shared or made available publically (Berazneva 2014; Speer and Stokoe 2014).

Effort was made to discuss social support and not to discuss any area of life or health that may cause distress. Women participants were also provided information about free counseling services from a trained psychologist if they required them. Two women belong to Pakistan, one is from Bangladesh, and the fourth is from India. A semi-structured qualitative questionnaire was used during data collection in order to provide better focus for the responses and discussion. However, women were free to discuss any part of their lived experiences and share whatever they wanted to beyond the semi-structured questions, as is inherent of qualitative research. There were seven questions in all and the objective was to enquire about: (i) the most prominent life challenges faced due to their health condition, (ii) the ways in which family and society supported them, and (iii) coping strategies to survive in society with chronic and permanent health conditions.

3.2 My Crime of Cancer

29 years old, Bangladesh

"People call me a cancer survivor, but I am not! I am a criminal. I have been sentenced to a never-ending punishment.

I got engaged at 19 and married two years later. Everything in my life was about marriage and children. However, nothing went as planned, as I was unable to conceive for two years. Tests for infertility eventually led to the discovery of cancer in my uterus.

When I went for cancer screening, the hospital staff gave me pep talks and counseling sessions. They handed me brochures about how to manage my life and reduce stress. But these brochures did not tell me how to manage my family and relatives.

A hysterectomy was done and after a year and half of treatment I was cancer-free. I thought my troubles were over.

What I didn't know was that my husband was waiting for my final tests and reports to share that he was taking a second wife. The world supported him. Even my parents understood. Everyone understood his duty to reproduce, and his generosity in not divorcing me when he took a second wife. The truth is he was able to start his life again, but mine was finished the day he took another wife!

Some relatives ask me why I do not return to my parents' house. Is it not obvious that I am not welcome in my parents' house as a "*talaq-shuda*" (divorcee) daughter? I am expected to be brave and patient and live for my parents' happiness. After all, Islam allows up to four marriages. But I have no peace. With the status of a regular wife and hope of having children taken away from me with my womb gone, I do not know the purpose of my life.

My world and attention revolves around my husband and news of his other wife and his newborn son. It would not be wrong if you call me a cybercriminal...I am constantly trying to track information about his life and marital state through Facebook. It may be that I am looking for evidence of something going wrong in their marriage? I hate this about myself, but I cannot stop.

I was a part-time teacher for a year, but during my treatment, I was turned away from the job and now when I reapply, as the school is walking distance from my home and the only convenient option for me to work at, they do not entertain my call or application.

A few years ago, I asked my father to send me abroad for studies if he cannot keep me in his home. But he refused, saying he does not have that kind of money. He stated: "Isn't it enough what all has happened to you, do you want to ruin your reputation further by travelling and living alone in a foreign land." The only escape from our culture and society is to leave. I dream of leaving one day.

My husband has never been mean to me, but what hurts is that he has a big family which gets together regularly, and he has now gotten used to not taking me. When I asked him he said that he doesn't want me to risk infection as my immunity is low due to my cancer history.

What hurts even more is that even my only sister hides things from me...she hid her trip to Turkey and the birthday party of her son.

I myself do not want to go anywhere even if invited. When I go out, I am asked about my health condition, routine annual tests, or my husband's remarriage. I prefer to stay at home and look after the house. My heart is broken, and I do not want to go sightseeing or go to weddings. I prefer the walls of my house and seclusion.

Allah brought me to this…and put me in this position. I have left my revenge in his hands. He will punish those who have hurt me…discarded me, and made my life more difficult than it is.

3.2.1 Analysis

It is evident that there are rigid social constructions of illness being associated with self-blame and guilt for women in South Asia. In this narration the woman believes that by getting cancer, she is paying for some sin that she has committed, by referring to herself as a "criminal." There is also a strong thread of parental rejection. Though parents are considered to be the "significant others" in terms of seeking refuge and providing support when conjugal bonds fail, in this story the parents have rejected their daughter. The narrator is unable to return to her parents home and has to accept a life with an inferior status of a second wife in her husband's house. This is possibly because parents in South Asia prefer for their daughters to retain their "wife" status, rather than assume a *divorcee* label (Parvez 2011).

One of the prominent themes revealed through this narration is that there is still excessive burden of reproduction and fertility on women of South Asia in order to secure their marriages and gain social status. Despite entering the millennium, South Asian women still face immense pressure to maintain marriages through reproduction or else suffer some form of permanent estrangement from husband, in this narration the estrangement being remarriage without permission from the first wife. The fact that a woman's marital identity and conjugal bond is primarily shaped by her fertility is acceptable not just by the husband's family, but also the parents of the narrator.

Unable to emerge from her status as a wife, the narrator is not able to find other options of occupation and engagement in life. The doors of employment have been closed, due to geographical immobility and lack of access to jobs in her vicinity. Her father has refused to provide her with opportunities for higher education from a foreign university to better her life opportunities and possibly provide her a means to escape from her present circumstances. Family and relatives support her husband in not integrating her in family events. In this way, the participant is bound by society's clutches and cannot escape her life as a discarded wife in her husband's house, forced to cyber-stalk her husband and his second wife. She awaits news that would perhaps alert her about problems between her husband and his second wife, and in this way the narrator not only likes herself less and is suffering from low self-esteem, but has another reason for considering herself a "criminal."

The woman participant shares how she is excluded from family gatherings and also in the sharing of family news. We are able to juxtapose the infertility label with the Hindu widow label in South Asian society. South Asian Hindu societies have historical traditions of excluding widows from social gatherings like weddings and births, as widows were considered ill-fated (Chen 1997). This narration suggests that South Asian society also fears the following two possibilities with regard to infertile women. First, that association with infertile women might bring ill fortune for other women, especially on auspicious days, almost like fertility is a contagious disease. Second, that the envy and internal despair of an infertile woman might hurt the lives of other women with children.

There is also a serious issue in South Asian healthcare services with regard to inadequacies in healthcare counseling support for chronic and terminal illnesses. Doctors insist on following international protocols of debriefing patients and providing them full information and diagnosis, without realizing that the emotional support from relatives and community is not the same in South Asia as it is in the West. Presently, there are no services for counseling the patient with consideration of life circumstances and support networks. Women of South Asia face challenges that necessitate the development of counseling protocols which are region specific and consider cultural and religious values and beliefs. The woman in this story believes that the community and culture cannot be changed and the only solution is to leave South Asian society and regain value in Western societies. It is evident that assumptions of lack of acceptance in native society contribute to great dissatisfaction and despair in the narrator. The inability of South Asian women to rebuild their lives or develop intimate relationships after failure of marriage or serious health problems is a concern. This may be a gender-specific problem, with men having health problems or handicaps not suffering from this kind of rejection and exclusion and still being considered marriage material (Hanna and Rogovsky 1991; Maya Dhungana 2006).

Finally, there is a disturbing and distressing theme of resentment and revenge. The woman in this story is profoundly hurt by the treatment of society after her cancer treatment and ultimate loss of fertility. Multiple sources of rejection faced by the woman participant have contributed to loss of dignity and autonomy, including: (i) the second marriage of her husband, (ii) refusal of her father to provide her an escape through higher education abroad, (iii) employment-led autonomy in the future, (iv) rejection of family and in-laws during family events, and (v) lack of culturally relevant support by healthcare practitioners and counselors. Her hurt is so deep that she is unable to forgive and mentions her need for "revenge." Unable to take revenge herself, she now awaits God to take revenge against all those who have hurt her, rejected her, and prevented her from resuming a new life after her treatment.

3.3 Paralyzed Spirits

50 years old, India

I was born with paralyzed legs. Despite repeated surgeries in my early years, this condition was irreversible. Though awareness of disability has increased ...there is still no social acceptance, especially for physically handicapped women. People see my disability, before they see me.

I became independent quite early despite my disability. Many women I know do far less than me. My first training at home was that my mother would leave me near the tap to wash the clothes with a soap bar. Slowly my mother added to my tasks. She would chop vegetables and meat and place it on the stove. I would then be responsible for stirring the *salan*[1] and taking it off from the stove when it was ready. With time I became a very good cook and even started a catering business. I can sweep the floors and do the dusting by moving around the house in my wheelchair.

I can easily say that for me, spending months in Pampers after surgery, and being bound to a wheelchair for life, has not been as painful as when my husband left me. I met and fell in love with a man who I thought would love me forever. I was pretty and young and willing to please him. There was no family present for my wedding, only our friends. I argued with my parents, left my house, took risks with my health and bones to be intimate with him.

After a few months of my marriage, I asked for money to buy something for my parents when I visited home. My husband didn't give me the money and instead initiated a fight and ended up slapping me. I decided after that never to ask him for money again. I realized he can beat me and I can never fight back or complain to anyone, so I learnt to protect myself from him by never asking him for anything. This became difficult for me as I was financially dependent on him. The special recipes I wanted to cook for him needed expensive ingredients that I could not ask him for.

I realize now that it was not him who was abusive, but it was the lack of acceptance by society which placed great strain on him. At first he was like a hero who had rescued a girl no one was willing to love or marry. It was all very romantic. But the realities of marriage, the inability to have children, and the sly comments and conspiracies of his family finally ruined our marriage. His mother and sisters would regularly say: "what a beautiful son/brother God has given us, and what *qismat*[2] he has that his wife is not a match for him."

It has been 15 years since our divorce, but I cannot forget or forgive. After two years of pleasing him, cooking for him, building a home with him, he said that he had decided to please his mother by going back to live with her as she was showing signs of old age and illness. I begged to go with him and swore that I would look after his mother better than any daughter-in-law could, but he insisted his mother would never accept me.

Eventually even the doors of my workplace closed on me. I had a very close friend who was a fellow teacher. We remained friends for more than ten years. One day out of the blue, she messaged me and said that she could not be my friend anymore, as it kept her trapped. She was unable to climb the stairs and sit in the staff room and make friends with others. I understood. After all, I sat downstairs in the

[1] *Salan* is a gravy made from meat or vegetables.

[2] "*Qismat*" translated to mean fate

accounts office and she had been giving me company for ten years without being able to enjoy the company of others. But it hurt so much. I felt rejected and discarded again.

A few months after this, I left my teaching job. I think my choice to leave had a lot to do with the rejection and loss of my friend. I know I should not have involved my ego and feelings and stayed for the sake of my students, but I just could not help it. I still have my food catering business and thank God I can do this from home and remain independent.

Over my life I have heard family and relatives say that: "She is suffering because of the sins of her parents." I don't believe that God is so cruel, that he created us like this at birth to punish us or our parents! Yet, I don't know what the Quran says about biological inadequacies and deformity. If there are verses of the Quran that ensure support and acceptance for us, then where are they? And why don't people talk about those verses in Friday prayers, instead of other things?

I have never needed more than what God has prevented me from having. I believe I was an asset for my parents and my ex-husband. If there were ramps everywhere and society changed their attitudes, people like me might be able to have a normal life...we could go to the cinema with family or to the park. Our lives would not be like they are now.

3.3.1 Analysis

This narration confirms that South Asian society sees disability and physical handicap before the individual. Despite the fact that this participant comes from an advantaged background, the people she is interacting with are measuring her worth not as a family member or a professional worker, but by her handicap. Sadly, even education has not enlightened many societies to consider that by measuring a woman's worth by her handicap and limiting her potential, society is collectively losing agency in the family and productivity in the economy. In this story we learn about the resilience, coping strategies, and the autonomy of the handicapped. Physical disability does not prevent women from fulfilling life responsibilities or remaining independent and active. However, women's activity and involvement is limited to the home and there is lesser acceptance for participation in the public sphere for physically disabled women.

There are rigid expectations of marriage in South Asian society. We know that the primary goal is reproduction, but there is also considerable pressure to marry wives that are physically acceptable to society and are also considered physically compatible with the husband. It is obvious in this narration that there is need for the broadening of social constructions of marriage to emphasize the importance of mental compatibility. The conjugal bond in South Asian society seems to be dependent on social approval and acceptance of physical compatibility, with little attention to emotional connection, intellectual rapport, or personality disposition.

It may be that the general culture of discrimination against the handicapped has licensed men to take advantage of physically disabled women in their youth. In this story, the woman participant feels that she has been used in her youth and later abandoned when not needed. Men are known to abandon women after their initial sexual urges have been fulfilled and there is nothing new left in the relationship in terms of physical and sexual gratification and also when illness starts interfering in marital life (Glantz et al. 2009; Ussher et al. 2015). Additionally, the lack of sponsorship and protection offered to handicapped women by society empowers men to abuse and impose violence against women without suffering social censure. It is also easier to abuse women who cannot hit back physically and cannot leave or complain to others.

This narration also reveals the polemic South Asian tendency for men to be exonerated from all blame, even when they discard their marriage vows. Instead blame is placed on other women for conspiracies leading to marital dissolution. We find that during her narration the participant romanticizes the past by claiming her husband left, not due to personal choice but instead due to pressure from his mother and sisters. Mothers and sisters are not supportive of their sons and brothers marrying women with permanent health problems, especially related to infertility or physical handicaps. This may be because the social status of a woman is irrevocably linked and associated with the reputation and status of their significant male members of the family. There is serious concern about women's solidarity and support for other women with disabilities, given that women are primary care providers in the home for the sick and handicapped people in South Asian societies.

We also find that the few women who resist social trends by befriending handicapped women in South Asian society are not able to maintain their support and patronage. They end up abandoning handicapped women due to the fatigue and exhaustion of being the only supporters in a society that does not have widespread social support. In this story, specific barriers to social integration and the development of social networks are shared, such as isolation from workplace common rooms and staff rooms and the lack of installation of ramps and lifts. In all, barriers to public spaces and workplaces lead to barriers for social capital development, as lack of physical access disempowers handicapped people from socializing and networking.

There is also confusion about religion and deformity. The punitive tendencies in South Asian culture still consider deformity to be a penance for a sin that either the woman herself has committed or her parents or family have committed. There is a complex theme of women being blamed and having to suffer for the sins of others in South Asian society. This is also evident in cultural practices which are usually sustained in the name of tradition and religion, such as the *watta satta*[3] system

[3] *Watta satta* refers to the custom of marrying one brother and sister in exchange for another brother and sister. The custom is associated with different forms of violence against women, such as reciprocal mistreatment, domestic violence, and divorce.

(Kavesh 2012), honor killing episodes, and *Jirga*[4] penalties of raping women as punishment for the crimes committed by their male kin (Iqbal 2007; Niaz 2013).

3.4 The Childless Care Provider

35 years old, Pakistan

When I was diagnosed with cancer after two years of marriage I thought my world had ended. Not only was I sent home to my father for treatment, but after my womb was removed due to hysterectomy, and it became obvious that I could never reproduce, the doors of my husband's house were closed on me forever.

That time of recovery from chemotherapy and radiation for me was a blur and my father coordinated the divorce paper work. I believed no greater stigma could touch me than being childless and being abandoned by my husband. But after five years of my divorce my father was detected with prostate cancer. Discovered at an advanced stage, I fought for five long years to provide him with the best palliative care and emotional support. After the initial months of his diagnosis, I started believing there was a reason for my tragedy and my husband's abandonment…I was meant to be with my father and to provide him with the care I could only have provided as an unmarried and childless woman. God had given my life a purpose.

However, again society broke me. As I became more in tune with my new role as a care provider and was able to bring the rest of the world into focus again; I began to comprehend the whispers and talk of relatives and society. Their opinions and judgments became louder in my ears and consciousness, until it has consumed my life and thought process. I heard people say repeatedly on different days and about my father and me: "she is such as '*bad-qismat*'[5] girl- not only is she '*be-aulad*'[6] and '*talaq-shuda*', but now her father is dying from cancer. He has to leave the world knowing there is no one to carry his name forward."

I cannot recount the pain society has put me through or the suffering.

What hurts the most, during my time in this world, since the day I was born, the shame of being a girl has never left me. This is something I can never live down. I wonder sometimes if this is what Islam is. It must be… as all of the people in the world who discriminate against girls seem to be Muslims. I feel like I am being punished by living this life and my father was punished by having a daughter. The ones loved by Allah have progeny, and the ones discarded by Allah are childless, like me.

[4] Jirga refers to a traditional or tribal council of leaders who pass verdicts based on traditions and customs or religious interpretation. *Jirga* laws are associated with different forms of violence against women such as beatings, forced marriages, and gang rape.

[5] "*Bad-qismat*" translates to mean ill-fated.

[6] "*Be-aulad*" translates to mean childless.

I heard a relative at my father's funeral say: "There is no one to carry on the name of Fahad Bhai*,[7] what a great tragedy." This is what mine and my father's life is reduced to…begetting lineage. What we did in our lives or how we treated others is all forgotten.

I spent every waking hour serving my father. Between medication, preparing food, feeding him, washing clothes and bedsheets and arranging money, I was told that I was unable to save my father because of my prayers and piety. There is not one relative or visitor who did not tell me: "Did you read the wazifa[8] correctly… did you complete all the requisite days of the wazifa…Allah only accepts the prayer if you do it correctly and with a pure heart." Society has left no stone unturned to make it obvious to me that my lack of piety resulted in my prayers not being answered for my own health and ability to have children, the continuation of my marriage, and also for the long healthy life and painless death of my father.

As if the strain of slowly losing my father everyday was not great enough, but my troubles were added to while I saw his reactions to the sale of assets, jewelry, and a small plot of land, for the finances needed for his health maintenance. He had collected these assets for me with a lot of hard work. I could see the pain and helplessness in his eyes. Every day that he stayed alive, he suffered even more because he believed he was taking away my security.

People believe in our region that if you visit the sick, you are earning *sawab.*[9] From my memories what makes me most angry is that I was unable to bar people from visiting my father during the five-year period when we were fighting to make him comfortable and keep him positive to fight his illness. An endless stream of insincere relatives would visit, just to tell my father he has only a few months to live or to ask him: "how do you feel knowing you have only a few months left?" Is this how people believe they earn *sawab* from Allah?

3.4.1 Analysis

We find again in this narration that there is a strong theme in South Asian society of relegating a woman's role in life to reproduction in marriage. The complex burden that women carry is that they must not only be biologically capable for reproduction to secure and retain their marriage but also in order to compensate for being born a daughter in their father's house. Not only do women have to secure their marriage by reproducing children, but they must also compensate their fathers by having children. For childless women, social redemption can never be gained, either in their husband's home or their father's. Needless to say, given the biological factors

[7] Name of father has been changed to preserve anonymity.

[8] Wazifa refers to the religious instruction or specific guidelines for how a prayer must be performed, usually in repetition and over a multiple number of days.

[9] *Sawab* means reward from Allah.

and lack of agency in influencing many causes of infertility, women suffer considerable despair and rejection when they are assigned blame and shame for the inability to reproduce.

We learn from this story that for a daughter who has no child or husband, to further be fated to lose a father through terminal illness is the last form of social disgrace. To be left in this world without a male guardian and to not have been able to provide her father with grandchildren is a social disgrace which this participant is unable to live down. This burden must be especially acute for daughters who are the only child in South Asian families. Not only has the woman in this case specifically lost her social status by becoming a divorcée, but she is further in disgrace due to the inability of securing lineage for her father. It is true that there is an identity crisis of South Asian woman since they are exclusively perceived as daughters, wives, or mothers and they do not have their own individual identity or standing in society. This is also evident in how the participant dedicates many years of her life to her father's care and neglects to build an identity for herself, perhaps through education and work participation, or travel and wider community service.

There is also grave social pressure on women to save their terminally ill relatives through their prayers and piety. Immeasurable pressure is placed on women through fallacious religious interpretations that diseases must be cured through spiritual associations. The labeling and stigmatization of women as "impious" by society, if their prayers are not answered, may have the effect of creating estrangement in women from religion and spirituality. This is unfortunate, as faith and worship can be a source of great support and solace for women who are otherwise facing social rejection and shaming (Ishara 2018; Rokach and Brock 1998). We find that the social status of South Asian women is not just linked to fertility and marriage, but it is also deeply linked to their perceived piety by society in assisting the recovery of ill relatives and their significant others. This may have roots in the widely prevalent South Asian cultural belief that daughters and wives are responsible for bringing prosperity and fortune in their father's and husband's lives. Consequently, this belief may invite weighty blame and liability on women when family circumstances turn unfortunate.

This narration also brings to life the known and critical lack of security net for women in South Asia, who are deprived of government sponsorship and support (Bano et al. 2009; Devereux 2001). Consequently, there is pressure on significant male relatives, like the father, brother, and husband, to leave assets, wealth, property, and jewelry to women for safeguarding their future. In this age when women of the world are gaining social rank due to their education and achieved status, South Asian women are still in need of family assets for their social status and security. Ultimately the social status of South Asian women is linked with their inheritance and wealth, with women who have more assets receiving greater status and acceptance, compared to those who do not have wealth. This may also be an important reason why female feticide and son preference are still very high in the region (Abrejo et al. 2009). The dilemma of leaving female relatives, like the daughter, sister, and wife, with adequate jewelry and property to provide them with security and status in society is not uncomplicated or trouble-free for men. This may also be a cause for many men preferring not to seek expensive healthcare as they do not want to die leaving their women dependents without assets and a security net. Another reason for the sustained deprioritization of education, and the more expensive higher education, for girls in South Asia is due to the expense. It is deemed more financially prudent to leave daughters with fixed assets and wealth than provide them with costly higher education.

3.5 The Blind Masseur

48 years old, Pakistan

I was born blind in a poor village. My father was a daily wage laborer and my mother never worked for money. There was no school for blind children in my village, and I received no formal education. Three of my elder sisters attended some years of schooling, but all three had left school by the time they were 8–9 years old. Hearing my sisters read or listening to TV has been the only education I have received.

I truly believe that there is no difference between me and the walls of my house…the bricks cannot read, and neither can I.

It is a twist of fate that the tragedy of me being born blind became my family's biggest asset; I earned more money in a week than even my father. There was a neighboring woman who came to our house when I was around 8 years old and told my mother: "she is Gods special child, I have intense pain in my head, if she touches it and reads a prayer, I will feel better." When I pressed her head and recited *Ayat-ul-Kursi*,[10] she declared with relief that she truly felt better. This was the beginning. I learnt to develop my *malish* (massage) skills, by practicing on family members and village women and remaining vigilant of their sounds of appreciation. I also continued to recite all the prayers my mother had been teaching me during the *malish* and this made me very popular.

By the age of 10, I was providing *malish* services in the community to most of the elderly women. They started repaying my mother…either in kind or in whatever little money they had. A few years later, after I had got my periods, my mother asked the local *Dai* (midwife) to train me to do the *Chila Malish*.[11] I soon became more popular than her and started earning consistent income for the family.

There were more *rishtas*[12] for me than for my seven sisters; five were elder than me. By 25 years I was married to a man who was 45 years old and had children my age. He paid my parents more than the other suitors for my hand in my marriage. I

[10] Ayat-ul-Kursi refers to a powerful prayer from Quran, which is read commonly for healing and protection.

[11] *Chila Malish* refers to the massage provided to a woman for 40 days after she gives birth. This is a tradition in South Asia which is culturally mandatory as it is believed that this massage will not only rejuvenate a woman to return to her domestic duties with complete health, but will also prepare her for another healthy pregnancy.

[12] *Rishta* refers to a marriage proposal.

was lucky that his first wife had died when he married me. He lived in the city and was also a daily wage earner like my father. Sometimes he earned as a painter and sometimes as a bricklayer.

After my marriage, many clients and neighbors told my husband to visit a clinic in the city to see if my vision could be restored, but my husband never took me for a checkup. I was more lucrative to him blind. People prefer blind *malish-walis*,[13] in a conservative society like ours. As I was young and healthy I was able to earn money during the day by serving five clients in one day. I also used to *malish* my husband in the night until he fell asleep. Naturally, I earned much more in the city than I did in my village. I found clients through word of mouth. Most of the women in my neighborhood worked as domestic helpers and they were kind enough to ask their female employers for work for me.

In the first five years of marriage I became a mother to three children, two sons and a daughter. My eldest, a son, was blind like me. For my son, my husband visited many doctors, but by Allah's will he remained blind.

I always believed my elder son would never leave me as he was blind like me. We were both illiterate and we understood each other like no one else did. Last year he got married and I asked his wife for only one thing, not to treat me like a mother-in-law, but a friend. But within three months of the marriage she had created rifts and fights and ultimately she left with my son. I cried for days until I became sick.

It was in *Ramadan*[14] that *Rasool Allah* (*saw*)[15] came in my dreams and convinced me to forget my elder son and only depend on Allah. Since then I do not cry for anyone or have any expectations from anyone. I only rely on Allah. But there is still this immense pain in my heart.

Now at this age I am a widow, with the greatest insecurity that someone can enter my house at night or that when I am old and sick there will be no way to earn money. I rarely sleep with a full stomach and I worry about the next day.

However, I am still grateful to Allah. I have a house of half a *Marla*.[16] Allah is my Keeper, and He is all I need...maybe these two (children) will also leave me one day, but I will still have Allah.

3.5.1 Analysis

There is a persistent social belief that it is acceptable not to send special needs people to school in South Asia. Furthermore, in this narration it is evident that women from poor and disadvantaged backgrounds have no access to the Braille

[13] *Malish-wali* refers to a woman who provides massage services.

[14] Ramandan is the month of the fasting in the Muslim calendar.

[15] *Rasool Allah* refers to Prophet Muhammad and *saw* means peace and blessings be upon the Prophet.

[16] Half a *Marla* refer to approximately 15 square yards.

education system. Although it is expected that Braille education is not available in rural areas of South Asia (Miles 2002), in this narration we find that even children born in the urban city are deprived of special needs education. This may be because of low public sector provision, inequalities in educational provision, and expensive or inaccessible private education (Unterhalter 2006).

Though the life of a permanently handicapped woman belonging to the lower wealth class is crippled by financial pressures and insecurity, she is still an asset for her relatives. We already know that South Asian society considers free domestic labor provided by women a right of all households, but we also find that physically handicapped women may have to share greater burdens of domestic labor compared to other women due to their restriction to the house. As a girl the woman in this narration is not only deprived of any form of education, formal or informal, but is used as the primary domestic laborer for a large family. The money that she earns from providing massage services goes to her household and family. What comes to the forefront in this story is that there is considerable exploitation of the handicapped for financial gain by parents and husband. In this case, the parents benefit from the handicapped daughter before marriage and the husband benefits after marriage. We may also have learnt from this story that there is an alternative to dowry in the form of assurance that the girl being given away in marriage can earn an income from paid employment.

We know that women in South Asia have strong social dependencies on men. Passed from their father's house to their husbands and then their sons, women are highly dependent on the patronage and protection of their male relatives. In this story the woman describes how she offered an olive branch to her daughter-in-law by requesting her not to treat her like a mother-in-law. Social constructions and traditions compel women to believe there will be problems in this relationship. Mother-in-laws across all societies of the world have bad social images, but this is more pronounced in South Asia because of the high dependency on men and the battle of women to control men. Mother in law and daughter in laws in South Asia especially have traditions of estrangement, violence, and crime (Rew et al. 2013; Vera-Sanso 1999).

After her son's abandonment, the participant turns to another male model, the Prophet of Islam, to find internal solace and comfort herself that at least she has a spiritual leader and God who will not abandon her. We also learn that religion is being used by the woman narrator to seek not just personal solace, but also social status and professional acceptance. She secures confidence in her clientele through reciting verses of the Quran and the special professional edge that she is providing to her clients is the combination of physical massage with spiritual healing. In this way, religion is a tool for the disadvantaged to gain social power. At the same time, we also learn about the contradictory mental trauma of needing religion but also having little faith. The woman in this narration swings between hope and uncertainty. At one moment in the interview she testifies to her strong faith in God and in the next describes her insecurity over her future stability. Similarly, she testifies to only needing God after her son's abandonment but also describes the aching void that cannot be filled just with religious faith. This confusion is the strongest indicator for the importance of the supportive role of society and family in the lives of women.

3.6 Conclusion

Needless to say, these subjective narrations cannot be generalized to the entire South Asian region. Yet, the stories carry important weight in describing lived realities of South Asian women who have health conditions related to chronic disease, terminal disease, or physical disability. There are considerable cultural barriers to ill and handicapped South Asian women gaining social acceptance and family approval. Apart from social stigma and exclusion, the absence of lifts and ramps become solid barriers for the disabled to participate in public spaces and enter or succeed at the workplace. Despite this, the narrations in this chapter highlight the strong agency of the four women. The first narrator is living as a discarded second wife in her husband's house, with no support from her parents. She has left her revenge to God and has assumed passivity and compliance. Not many women would survive such an existence. The second has learned to perform all domestic chores as a paraplegic from a young age including cleaning, cooking, and washing. She has been a teacher and is currently catering food as a home-based worker. As a cancer survivor and an abandoned wife, the third narrator became a tireless care provider for her terminally ill father, which must have required great physical and emotional stamina. The last narrator has been the primary income earner in her household since childhood despite being blind and illiterate. Now as a widow she is the primary earner for her children and as an informal worker must learn to survive through her aging years without a provident fund or pension net.

We find that South Asian women who suffer health challenges accept considerable blame and that this is a cultural and traditional norm in patriarchal and punitive South Asian societies. The use of language to describe themselves as *sinners* or *criminals* highlights the plight of women in pulling themselves into a void of guilt and censure and further indicates that such women must suffer great emotional and mental health turmoil through their lives as a consequence of punitive social labeling. Marriage for South Asian women is still exclusively associated with reproduction and fertility. Women who cannot beget lineage are discarded by husbands and in-laws, sustaining a society that values and ranks women based on biological fecundity over personage. As women believe their roles to be limited to marriage and motherhood, due to social conditioning from birth, they are unable to create an identity for themselves as single and childless women in South Asian society. There is also the social problem of physical beauty being considered a necessary condition for the complete woman in South Asia. Thus, women who have physical handicaps are discriminated in society and not considered marriage material in a region where arranged marriages are the norm. Oppressive societal labels of "*talaq-shuda*" (divorcee), "*Be-aulad*" (childless), and "*Bad-qismat*" (ill-fated) also contribute to shaming and exclusion of women who face health challenges and infertility. We found an interesting but unfortunate juxtaposition, in the case of infertile women of South Asia suffering similar shame and social exclusion that Hindu widows have historically experienced in the region. Superstitious fears of infertile women causing similar ill-fate in other women of society compel people to exclude women from their conversations and family events, causing greater pain and isolation in childless women.

Different themes emerge with regard to parental support for South Asian women suffering from health problems and marital abandonment. There is a middle-class father who is unwilling to support and fund his daughter for higher education, even though this would enable her to escape from her second wife status as a shamed and discarded wife. In another narration a paraplegic woman does not receive support from her parents for her marriage and this may be one of the reasons for the abuse and easy abandonment she faced in her marriage. Parental support may have ensured greater social respect and marital stability, as husbands and in-laws would face pressure to behave with restraint. In another narration a father who is terminally ill and requires money for expensive health costs is pained deeply that his illness is responsible for depleting the assets he had planned to leave for his daughter. Not only is there great burden on South Asian families to leave a significant asset base for their daughter highlighted, but the emotions and helplessness of the father is a source to exacerbate the pain and agony for the grieving daughter. Impoverished parents are found to benefit from the work and income of their blind daughter from an early age. They do not have the resources and awareness to invest in the health or education of their blind daughter. Later they choose a husband for their daughter based on who will pay the most for her hand in marriage and do not consider the age gap or compatibility of their daughter.

We find two interesting but unfortunate themes related to father and daughters in South Asia. First, those daughters also carry burden of begetting lineage for fathers, and not just husbands, in order to compensate for being born a daughter. Second, there is immense pressure on fathers to build and leave behind a security net for their daughters. This security net may include land, property, jewelry, and other assets. Findings imply that society and traditions sustain the reduced status of daughters in South Asia. Culturally, a father who has nothing to leave his daughter faces guilt and shame. Similarly, social constructions are shaped to make daughters who are unmarried and without children to feel unworthy and insignificant. Though physical abuse and violence by husbands is a norm in South Asia, abuse against physically handicapped and ill women is a reality less understood. One of the reasons why abuse against disabled women might be very high is because spouses do not expect a response or attempt to escape from victims who are immobile and dependent because of their physical handicap. We find in our narrations that men are exonerated for blame and instead women in-laws are usually blamed for inciting the men, namely, mother-in-laws and sister-in-laws. Here we feel there may be an opportunity to raise awareness about the reasons for women's lack of support for each other. Women's status is irrevocably linked to that of their male relatives. Thus, women who are abusing other women are doing so due to a complex web of insecurities and dependencies. We propose that social awareness and media be used to promote gender solidarity and support for disabled and ill women.

There is despair in the adoption of Western or International protocols for counseling and care practices for women patients. Development of protocols and counseling with a region-specific focus is important as it would recognize the cultural circumstances and challenges of women patients. We recommend that healthcare protocols in the region for counseling are developed in consideration of cultural realities in order to be more effective. Support groups need to recognize that women in South Asia are in need of help in dealing with the tangible and experienced circumstances caused by society. There needs to be considerable awareness and mobilization for regressive cultural practices which prevent women from emerging from their secondary status, including: (i) second marriage in the case of infertility, (ii) isolation and segregation of physically disabled and infertile women, and (iii) shaming of women who suffer from chronic disease and illnesses like cancer. This is possible through the combined efforts of legitimate religious scholars, media awareness campaigns, social media, television and cinema mediums, family counseling, and efforts by community notables. A considerable worry for South Asian communities is that women who are unable to take the reins of their own life or resume normal and complete lives after disease burdens feel so helpless and bitter that they are awaiting justice through the hands of God. Lack of forgiveness and inability to forget are noticeable themes in these stories, and they may be a cause for feelings of anger and mental instability in women.

The mental health and emotional stability of women who are facing insecurity and social isolation is being dealt with in extremely unhealthy ways including desire and hope for revenge at the hands of God. Given that women are also primary care providers in the homes and responsible for nurturing of children, emotional instability and feelings of anger in women would also have negative impact on other members of the family. There is also the attempt to compensate the deep loss of self-esteem caused by disease, disability, and infertility by using religion in different ways. The blind masseur is using religion to gain social power and professional status. The childless care provider is trying to use religion to secure health recovery for her father, but she is shamed and humiliated as nature and disease take her father's life eventually despite her prayers and devotion. Here, we learn of the great piety burden placed on women, who are humiliated and labeled *impious* when their prayers are not answered. Thus we find that not only is religious misinterpretation promoting a punitive culture for blaming women for deformity and ill-health, but it also places great burden on women for illness in their family members.

Finally, we find that it is believed by women that society will not change. One woman strongly believed that escape is only possible if she shifts to the West. Given that all the women of South Asia cannot shift countries, we recommend some changes in South Asian society at both cultural and state level, such as: (i) improved awareness and state subsidization for special needs girls and women; (ii) primary to higher educational access for special needs girls, and adult literacy and skill development for special needs women, and opportunities for home schooling and online learning; (iii) longitudinal assessment of special needs and disability; (iv) home-based work opportunities for disabled women and also women undergoing long-term health recovery plans; (v) improving social acceptance and participation in public spaces to raise acceptance and awareness; (vi) clarification of religious stance on infertility, disease, and women's status; (vii) attempt through media to change patterns in mother-in-law and daughter-in-law relationships, and introducing campaigns to improve women's solidarity and patronage; (viii) counseling protocols for women patients which must not follow international protocols, but rather be developed locally; (ix) changing social construction of marriage, conjugal bonds, reproduction, and dependency on men; (x) raising awareness and social work monitoring within the homes for the financial and sexual exploitation of ill and handicapped women; and (xi) altering punitive culture against women for ill-health, infertility, and even ill-health of male relatives.

References

Abrejo, F. G., Shaikh, B. T., & Rizvi, N. (2009). 'And they kill me, only because I am a girl'... a review of sex-selective abortions in South Asia. *The European Journal of Contraception Reproductive Health Care, 14*(1), 10–16.

Andrews, D., Nonnecke, B., & Preece, J. (2007). *Conducting research on the internet: Online survey design, development and implementation guidelines.*

Bano, S., Balzani, M., Siddiqui, H., Sharma, K., Wilson, A., Mitra, T., . . . Kelly, L. (2009). *Violence against women in South Asian communities: Issues for policy and practice*. Jessica Kingsley Publishers.

Berazneva, J. (2014). Audio recording of household interviews to ensure data quality. *Journal of International Development, 26*(2), 290–296.

Chen, M. A. (1997). Listening to widows in rural India. *Women: A cultural review, 8*(3), 311–318.

Devereux, S. (2001). Livelihood insecurity and social protection: A re-emerging issue in rural development. *Development policy review, 19*(4), 507–519.

Elgesem, D. (2015). Consent and information–ethical considerations when conducting research on social media. In *Internet Research Ethics* (pp. 14–34). Oslo: Cappelen Damm Akademisk.

Glantz, M. J., Chamberlain, M. C., Liu, Q., Hsieh, C. C., Edwards, K. R., Van Horn, A., & Recht, L. (2009). Gender disparity in the rate of partner abandonment in patients with serious medical illness. *Cancer, 115*(22), 5237–5242.

Hanna, W. J., & Rogovsky, B. (1991). Women with disabilities: Two handicaps plus. *Disability, Handicap Society, 6*(1), 49–63.

Hewson, C. (2003). Conducting research on the internet. *PSYCHOLOGIST-LEICESTER, 16*(6), 290–293.

Iqbal, N. (2007). Legal pluralism in Pakistan and its implications on women's rights. *Scratching the Surface: Democracy, Traditions, Gender, 101.*

Ishara, M. (2018). *Women, religion and spirituality in South Asia "one does not have to be a man in the quest of truth".*

Kavesh, M. A. (2012). On exchange marriage: "Wata sata" marriages in southern Punjab, Pakistan. *Indian Anthropologist, 42*, 35–50.

Mauthner, N. S., & Doucet, A. J. S. (2003). Reflexive accounts and accounts of reflexivity in qualitative data analysis. *Sociology, 37*(3), 413–431.

Maya Dhungana, B. (2006). The lives of disabled women in Nepal: Vulnerability without support. *Disability Society, 21*(2), 133–146.

Miles, M. (2002). Disability in South Asia-millennium to millennium. *Journal of Religion, Disability Health, 6*(2–3), 109–115.
Niaz, U. (2013). Violence against women in South Asia. In *Violence against women and mental health* (Vol. 178, pp. 38–53): Karger Publishers.
Parvez, K. N. (2011). *Social changes and women-initiated divorce in Dhaka, Bangladesh: Gaining or loosing power?* Bergen: The University of Bergen.
Polkinghorne, D. E. (2005). Language and meaning: Data collection in qualitative research. *Journal of Counseling Psychology, 52*(2), 137.
Rew, M., Gangoli, G., & Gill, A. K. (2013). Violence between female in-laws in India. *Journal of International Women's Studies, 14*(1), 147–160.
Rokach, A., & Brock, H. (1998). Coping with loneliness. *The Journal of Psychology, 132*(1), 107–127.
Speer, S. A., & Stokoe, E. (2014). Ethics in action: Consent-gaining interactions and implications for research practice. *British Journal of Social Psychology, 53*(1), 54–73.
Tausig, J. E., & Freeman, E. W. (1988). The next best thing to being there: Conducting the clinical research interview by telephone. *American Journal of Orthopsychiatry, 58*(3), 418–427.
Unterhalter, E. (2006). *Measuring gender inequality in education in South Asia*. Citeseer.
Ussher, J. M., Perz, J., & Gilbert, E. (2015). Perceived causes and consequences of sexual changes after cancer for women and men: A mixed method study. *BMC Cancer, 15*(1), 268.
Vera-Sanso, P. (1999). Dominant daughters-in-law and submissive mothers-in-law? Co-operation and conflict in South India. *Journal of the Royal Anthropological Institute, 5*(4), 577–593.

Chapter 4
Women's Role in Decision-Making for Health care in South Asia

Sara Rizvi Jafree, Rubeena Zakar, and Shaheda Anwar

4.1 Introduction

The ranking for South Asian countries for gender inequality is not favorable (Leopold et al. 2016). Gender inequality is measured by assessing key variables such as maternal mortality, adolescent birth rate, share of parliamentary seats, access to secondary education, and labor force participation. From a total of 189 countries, Bangladesh ranks at 136, India at 130, and Pakistan at 150. In South Asia's case, women's unfavorable health indicators are not because of biomedical causes or health service shortfalls, as much as they are because of sociocultural factors. There are behaviors within the community and household which still prevent women from accessing health and adopting optimal health behaviors in South Asia. The two health indicators of maternal mortality and adolescent birth rates are dismal for all three countries, and the predominant reason is sociocultural factors sustaining reproductive pressure with high rates of births by women aged 15–19 years (Akseer et al. 2017; Singh et al. 2016). Gender inequality statistics also highlight low literacy, low retention, and low enrollment in school of girls, which means lower overall health literacy and incapability to take decisions for health during adult years (Sheikh and Loney 2018). Low labor participation and over-hiring in the informal sector of women in South Asia also imply lack of health benefits from employment sector.

S. R. Jafree
Department of Sociology, Forman Christian College University, Lahore, Pakistan

R. Zakar
Institute of Social and Cultural Studies, University of the Punjab, Lahore, Pakistan

S. Anwar (✉)
Department of Microbiology, Bangabandhu Sheikh Mujib Medical University, Dhaka, Bangladesh

S. R. Jafree (ed.), *The Sociology of South Asian Women's Health*,
https://doi.org/10.1007/978-3-030-50204-1_4

Independent decision-making is a salient factor in determining women's overall quality of life and standard of living (Desai and Johnson 2005). It is common to measure women's decision-making through variables of "choice in marriage," "literacy," and "employment"; however, the variable of "decision-making for health" has been less researched and emphasized (Sathar and Kazi 2000). Once it is ascertained that women are educated and employed, it is derivatively believed that they are also able to exercise autonomous health decision-making. However, what we fail to consider is that access to education and employment is influenced by a combination of social obligations, state laws, and financial necessities. In this way, even when women are not health decision-makers, they may still have better access options for education and employment. The complexity of health decision-making is that it is still considered a private domain. The reproductive health of women and maternal mortality rates are influenced significantly by the health decision-making power of women. This decision-making power is socially allocated to South Asian women much before they get married and start reproducing. We must abandon the simplistic and deterministic assumption that only prenatal and postnatal health of women has an impact on maternal mortality rates and survival of child. Reproductive health is also impacted by numerous social factors that influence a woman from the day that she is born, such as her nutritional provision, her share for domestic duties as a growing girl, the amount of sunlight and physical exercise she is encouraged to get, her access to education and employment, and her socialization or social conditioning about her self-worth and health rights (Godha et al. 2013; Mumtaz and Salway 2009; Senarath and Gunawardena 2009).

Education and employment are factors that improve a women's capacity to control resources and her ability to assume rights for health decision-making. Gender gap in economic well-being and professional status are important factors to be considered. In rural Bangladesh, it was found that women from richer households sought more healthcare compared with those from poor households (Senarath and Gunawardena 2009). At the same time, there is also empirical evidence from South Asia which suggests that women's education and work participation may still not promote independent decisions for health (Jejeebhoy and Sathar 2001). Many educated and working women do not opt for institutional deliveries or trained healthcare practitioners. Why is this? The main reason is the type of education and employment. Women with partial literacy or secular education and women working in the informal sector of the economy do not gain autonomy. It may also be that educated and working women who fear being shunned, stigmatized, and labeled a "rebel" for assuming health rights independently do not choose to take autonomous health decisions. Independence in South Asian women requires great courage, fortitude, and emotional strength, and ironically, women might face more health problems after assuming rights for independent health decisions. This chapter will discuss the factors that are associated with independent health decision-making power of women of reproductive years in South Asia.

4.2 Demographic Health Surveys: Bangladesh, India, and Pakistan

For this chapter, we are using the most recently accessible datasets of Demographic Health Surveys (DHS) from Bangladesh (2014–2015), India (2015–2016), and Pakistan (2017–2018). Datasets from the same year were not available from these countries, and thus, the latest available data was used. DHS collects nationwide data on women of reproductive years, from age group 15–49 years. The number of women sampled across the three countries in each DHS includes Bangladesh, N = 17,863; India, N = 699,686; and Pakistan, N = 12,364. We aimed to find significant associations for decision-making for health in women of South Asia. P-value was calculated on the basis of chi-square statistics. For our analysis, we have taken ten independent variables of (1) age, (2) urban/rural belonging, (3) literacy, (4) wealth index, (5) total children born, (6) occupation, (7) type of earning, (8) watching TV, (9) health card for child immunization, and (10) justification for wife beating. We have applied cross tabulations on SPSS using the dependent variable of "decision-making for health." There are six response categories for "decision-making for health," including: (1) "Respondent alone," (2) "Respondent and husband/partner," (3) "Respondent and other person," (4) "Husband/partner alone," (5) "Someone else," and (6) "Other." We have compounded these six categories into three categories for analysis purposes, merging categories 2–3 into one category to denote "joint" decision-making and merging categories 4–6 into one category to denote when "others" are making health decisions for women.

Though some analysts may interpret joint decision-making favorably, we feel this result must be read with caution. When interpreting results for "joint" decision-making, we must consider that the role of family, husband, and in-laws is not so simple, in that women may actually not be involved in the final decision. Many South Asian women may prefer to portray their husband and family as supportive, by indicating "joint" decision-making in survey responses, as they perceive this to be a matter of family honor and loyalty (Marphatia et al. 2017). Even when women are given options for joint decision-making by relatives, they may opt to let their men and family decide health matters for them as dutiful wives and daughters. Similarly, dutiful women may allow their in-laws, and specifically their mother-in-law, to make decisions for them out of a sense of obligation and expectation of reward through amicability in the home and their acceptance in the home. Pleasing the in-laws and mother-in-law is a major concern for many women who do not want to be marginalized in a joint family arrangement and who desire to develop a support system to prevent spousal rejection (Allendorf 2017).

DHS is countrywide data and has the benefits of random sampling, thus assuring generalizability and external validity of findings. Generally, the limitations of survey research are widely understood in terms of recall bias, interviewer bias, and missing variables, but in addition, there are also problems in collecting data from the conservative and subjugated South Asian woman (Senarath and Gunawardena 2009). Women with multiple tasks, role burden, and anxiety of sharing personal information related to family and health may not share as comprehensively, as their research ethics would conflict with their personal ethics of time and loyalty to family. There is also the problem of DHS data not being consistently or comparatively collected across South Asian states, and thus, differences across nations might be a result of time differences. Though results from the three countries will be presented, we will not be focusing on explaining differences in results between countries because of the difference in dates of DHS results between countries. It is to be noted that all women in the sample have been included in the cross tabulation results, as this question of decision-making has been asked from all women and not just married women. Also, some of the frequencies do not match or add up to the total sample, due to missing data or incomplete responses. Percentage results have been presented in order to make the interpretation easier for readers. It must also be noted that some categories for variables have not been filled comparatively across countries. To take an example, for the variable "occupation," Bangladesh does not have data under the clerical category. This is one of the reasons why not many variables could be included in our final analysis and advanced regression tests could not be run on the datasets.

4.2.1 Sociodemographic and Health Characteristics of Women

Table 4.1 presents the sociodemographic and health characteristics of South Asian women of reproductive age 15–49 years, including Bangladesh, India, and Pakistan. Comparative results reveal that an overwhelming majority of women of reproductive age in South Asia cannot make health decisions alone: 85.0% from Bangladesh, 89.1% from India, and 92.7% from Pakistan. Less than 15% of women in all three countries can make health decisions independently, with Pakistan lagging behind at 7.3%.

Table 4.2 presents descriptive results for women who are able to make health decisions alone, jointly, or not at all, according to sociodemographic characteristics. Chi-square results are also presented to show the likelihood of association between the dependent and independent variables. The high p-value of all the results <0.000 reveals the goodness of fit in that health decision-making is significantly associated with sociodemographic variables of women. With regard to age, results show that a significant number of younger women between the ages of 15 and 29 years are

Table 4.1 Descriptive statistics for South Asian women's autonomy versus dependency, on family, husband, and in-laws, for decision-making in health

Country	Bangladesh			India			Pakistan		
Category	Alone	Joint	Other	Alone	Joint	Other	Alone	Joint	Other
Frequency (percentage)	2530 (15.0%)	8114 (48.2%)	6185 (36.8%)	9483 (10.9%)	56,238 (64.8%)	21,135 (24.3%)	914 (7.3%)	4.489 (35.7%)	7163 (57.0%)

Source: Data for this table has been retrieved from publically available datasets of the Demographic Health Surveys of Bangladesh (2014–2015), India (2015–2016), and Pakistan (2017–2018)

Table 4.2 Descriptive statistics and chi-square results for South Asian women's autonomy versus dependency for decision-making in health

Country	Bangladesh				India				Pakistan			
Category/variable	Alone %	Joint %	Other %	*P*- value	Alone %	Joint %	Other %	*P*- value	Alone %	Joint %	Other %	*P*- value
Age												
15–19	05.8	09.4	17.4	0.000	02.0	02.8	05.2	0.000	02.0	01.8	04.0	0.000
20–24	13.8	18.1	20.7		10.8	14.2	18.8		15.1	16.8	22.3	
25–29	20.0	19.7	18.1		17.9	19.9	21.5		30.5	30.9	32.2	
30–34	19.8	18.2	14.6		18.6	18.7	17.3		28.7	28.5	21.9	
35–39	16.9	13.6	10.5		19.0	17.1	14.7		16.7	15.9	14.1	
40–44	13.8	11.9	09.9		16.2	14.3	11.7		05.6	04.7	04.0	
45–49	10.0	09.1	08.9		15.6	13.0	10.8		01.4	01.3	01.5	
Literacy												
No education	22.5	21.8	22.3	0.000	32.8	31.8	37.1	0.000	36.3	41.0	59.8	0.000
Primary	28.9	28.7	30.0		14.9	14.2	14.5		14.7	13.6	13.3	
Secondary	38.0	38.4	39.6		42.0	43.8	41.3		28.2	24.5	17.4	
Higher	10.6	11.1	08.1		10.3	10.2	07.1		20.8	20.9	09.5	
Residence												
Urban	37.7	35.4	30.9	0.000	30.8	28.5	25.9	0.000	51.9	48.2	40.7	0.000
Rural	62.3	64.6	69.1		65.7	67.9	69.5		48.1	51.8	59.3	
Wealth index												
Poorest	14.2	17.4	20.2	0.000	16.5	17.6	20.3	0.000	14.9	20.0	25.7	0.000
Poorer	15.0	19.2	20.0		20.1	20.6	22.2		20.2	20.0	25.0	
Middle	19.8	20.0	21.0		21.1	20.9	21.3		21.4	19.8	19.6	
Richer	25.6	20.3	20.3		21.5	20.3	19.3		20.8	18.0	16.5	
Richest	25.4	23.1	18.5		20.8	20.6	16.9		22.6	22.1	13.2	
Total children												
None	05.7	08.0	14.2	0.000	07.3	08.8	12.8	0.000	12.0	11.4	13.1	0.000

(continued)

Table 4.2 (continued)

Country	Bangladesh				India				Pakistan			
Category/variable	Alone %	Joint %	Other %	*P*- value	Alone %	Joint %	Other %	*P*- value	Alone %	Joint %	Other %	*P*- value
1–2 children	47.7	50.4	47.6		48.0	48.6	46.8		22.1	23.6	22.8	
3–4 children	33.4	30.0	26.3		32.8	31.5	29.7		37.1	37.7	34.1	
5-6 children	10.6	09.2	08.9		09.2	08.5	08.0		17.6	18.0	17.1	
7 or more children	02.5	02.4	02.9		02.7	02.6	02.7		11.1	09.2	12.8	
Occupation												
Not working	62.5	65.7	72.2	0.000	60.8	68.7	74.2	0.000	82.4	82.5	90.3	0.000
Professional	03.7	03.1	01.1		03.4	02.7	01.4		04.6	04.2	01.4	
Clerical	–	–	–		00.6	00.3	00.2		00.5	00.0	00.0	
Sales	02.8	02.8	02.2		02.2	01.5	01.0		00.7	00.3	00.3	
Agriculture – self	01.0	01.3	00.8		–	–	–		03.3	04.4	03.1	
Agriculture – employed	12.3	14.0	13.9		18.3	16.5	15.8		–	–	–	
Domestic work	04.2	02.1	01.3		04.9	03.2	02.3		–	–	–	
Services	03.1	02.7	01.8		–	–	–		02.3	01.7	00.9	
Skilled manual	10.2	08.2	06.5		–	–	–		05.2	05.9	03.7	
Unskilled manual	00.3	00.1	00.1		07.9	06.0	04.3		–	–	–	
Type of earnings												
Not paid	06.1	07.1	10.3	0.000	14.9	20.7	23.9	0.000	07.4	06.4	15.2	0.000
Cash only	87.6	85.2	84.2		72.5	65.3	59.1		89.6	89.3	75.5	
Cash and in kind	05.0	06.6	04.0		08.9	09.9	10.5		00.6	02.4	04.7	
In kind only	01.3	01.2	01.5		03.7	04.1	06.4		02.5	01.9	04.6	
Watch television												
No	33.4	38.0	43.1	0.000	23.4	23.5	29.3	0.000	31.9	33.5	54.5	0.000
More than once a week	09.2	08.3	08.6		06.7	07.7	07.4		10.7	12.4	09.4	
Once a week or more	57.4	53.6	48.3		11.4	11.5	11.1		57.3	54.1	36.2	
Almost everyday	–	–	–		58.5	57.3	52.2		–	–	–	

Country	Bangladesh				India				Pakistan			
Category/variable	Alone %	Joint %	Other %	*P*- value	Alone %	Joint %	Other %	*P*- value	Alone %	Joint %	Other %	*P*- value
Health card												
No card	03.3	05.7	08.1	0.000	08.8	08.3	09.5	0.000	13.5	14.1	28.5	0.000
Yes, seen	61.6	65.6	64.6		59.7	60.5	57.3		59.6	58.1	50.8	
Yes, not seen	32.3	26.2	25.4		20.5	22.1	23.5		07.3	06.4	04.0	
No longer has card	02.8	02.5	01.9		11.0	09.2	09.7		19.6	21.4	16.6	
Beating justified												
No	77.7	82.0	75.6	0.000	70.2	73.5	66.7	0.000	64.4	74.9	47.9	0.000
Yes	21.9	17.7	23.9		28.9	25.9	32.6		33.3	23.3	49.9	
Don't know	00.4	00.2	00.5		00.9	00.7	00.7		02.3	01.9	02.2	

Source: Data for this table has been retriesved from publically available datasets of the Demographic Health Surveys of Bangladesh (2014–2015), India (2015–2016), and Pakistan (2017–2018)

unable to make decisions themselves (Bangladesh = 56.2%, India = 45.5%, and Pakistan = 58.5%). Pakistan ranks the worst in terms of women of reproductive years having no literacy at 51.4%, with India and Bangladesh following at 33.2% and 22.1%, respectively. Low literacy in South Asian women also implies low health literacy and health awareness in women, which prevents them from making health decisions that are favorable for both self and children. Figures for South Asian women with higher education are also very low, at less than 14% for Pakistan and less than 10% for Bangladesh and India. Nearly all the women across the three countries who are illiterate and with primary or secondary education have their health decisions made by others (Bangladesh = 91.9%; India = 92.9%; Pakistan = 90.5%).

A majority of women, between 55% and 68%, across all three countries reside in the rural areas. Most of these rural women have their health decisions made by "others" (Bangladesh = 69.1%; India = 69.5%; Pakistan = 59.3%). The plight of South Asian rural women is that they face critical problems related to healthcare access and quality due to underdevelopment and remoteness. Not only are healthcare centers and trained practitioners not available, but also South Asian rural areas are known for feudal and tribal patriarchy which prevent decision-making autonomy in women. A majority of women of reproductive age belong to the poor, poorest, or middle wealth class in all three countries, from 57% to 66%. Similarly, a majority of women from the poor and middle classes are unable to make their health decisions independently or jointly (Bangladesh = 61.2%; India = 63.8%; Pakistan = 70.3%). Our results show that in the absence of public sector health coverage or quality public health services in South Asia, women may be suffering from the dual burden of poverty and disease. As a compounding problem, we must also recognize that poorer women of South Asia face complex problems related to lack of education, opportunities for paid employment, and subsequent loss of social status and decision-making power.

Considerable numbers of South Asian women have more than three children (64.6% from Pakistan, 42.2% from India, and 41.1% from Bangladesh), implying social pressure to reproduce and have multiple number of children in South Asia. In Bangladesh and India, majority of women with no children or less than two children have their health decisions made by others (61.8% and 59.6%), with women in Pakistan following at near majority of 35.9%. Our results imply that women with fewer children in South Asia face greater control over their health decision-making, due to cultural and religious factors which compel family and in-laws to control their reproduction and birth spacing. A majority of women in all three countries are not working, with 86.9% from Pakistan, 69.2% from India, and 67.6% from Bangladesh. The predominant occupation for women is agricultural work and unskilled employment in the gray or informal economy in all three countries. Thus, we must consider that both the unemployed and those working in the informal sector have less health security. The latter is due to temporary contracts, irregular income, no provision for paid leaves during illness, lack of health insurance, and absence of pension or provident fund for old age health security. Nearly all women who are not working or working in the informal sector – agriculture, domestic service, and unskilled work – have their health decisions made by others (Bangladesh = 88.3%; India = 96.6%; Pakistan = 93.4%). A significant number of the working women are not being paid at all or are being paid in kind (20.6% from India, 10.2% from Pakistan, and 7.9% from Bangladesh). Many South Asian women working in unskilled or domestic services are paid in kind, through the provision of food or free accommodation in exchange for their work. Majority of working women who are being paid in cash, despite their independent income, are having their health decisions made by others (Bangladesh = 84.2%; India = 59.1%; Pakistan = 75.5%).

A significant number of women in South Asia have indicated that they have no exposure at all to television (45.3% from Pakistan, 39.2% from Bangladesh, and 24.9% from India). Those who have indicated watching TV are also unable to make health decisions independently or jointly (Bangladesh = 56.9%; India = 70.7%; Pakistan = 45.6%). This result just shows that the role of media in promoting autonomous decision-making in women is not materializing. Any health-related information imparted through television media in South Asia is not having a hypodermic syringe effect or even a slow-drip effect on women's health behavior for self and child or on family decision to allow autonomous decision-making in women. A significant number of women in all three countries do not have a health vaccination card for their child (ren), or have indicated that they have not seen it or no longer have it (35.3% for Bangladesh, 40.4% for India, and 46.1% for Pakistan). Nearly all the women who "have a health card" or "ever had a health card" do not have control over their health decision-making (Bangladesh = 91.9%; India = 90.5%; Pakistan = 71.4%). Decision for vaccination of children in South Asia is controlled by the husband and in-laws, as vaccinations are still believed to be Western vehicles to prevent fertility and sterility in future generations. Results for the health card also imply that perhaps South Asian mothers are still not aware about the importance of vaccination, due to cultural and religious factors influencing belief that vaccinations are harmful.

A significant number of women in Pakistan, India, and Bangladesh at 39.1%, 27.8%, and 20.6%, respectively, believe that beating by husband is justified. This is an extremely unfortunate result and suggests that women who believe it is justified to be physically abused based on matters such as bad cooking, inadequate childcare, and disagreement with husband and in-laws would also have low self-esteem and self-worth in assuming rights for decision-making. The results suggest that women believe it is justified to be physically abused based on matters such as bad cooking, inadequate childcare, or disagreement with husband and in-laws. The implications are grave, as women who believe they can be hit and abused would also passively accept other forms of invisible abuse, such as deprivation of rights for autonomous health decision-making. Additionally, such women would also have very low self-esteem and thus accept other forms of abuse and neglect, such as rights for leisure time, self-care, nutritional needs, education, and paid employment. This belief system of accepting violence by spouse and family is predominantly influenced by religious interpretations and endemic cultural traditions in all three countries. A significant number of women across all three countries who do not believe that there husband has a right to beat them have their health decisions made for them by others (Bangladesh = 75.6%; India = 66.7%; Pakistan = 47.9%). These results imply that women who have beliefs against patriarchal norms and women who resist violence face more control for health decision-making, as they are perceived by their families and in-laws to be nonconformists who require more control and regulation.

4.3 Discussion

We continue this chapter by discussing the most prominent sociocultural factors sustaining barriers to independent health decision-making in women of South Asia. This discussion will help in explaining the DHS results presented above and also in understanding the resilient social fabric which compels society and women to adopt or not adopt optimal health behaviors and assume or not assume health decision-making. The discussion includes five broad themes of: (i) gender gaps and family factors, (ii) health education and health behavior, (iii) nature of employment, (iv) violence and safety, and (v) quality of healthcare services and traditional healers.

4.3.1 Gender Gaps and Family Factors

Permission from Husband and In-Laws

The nature of the family has significant influence on the ability of women to make autonomous health decisions in South Asia (Lee and Beatty 2002; Wusu and Isiugo-Abanihe 2003). Women living in a joint family with in-laws have less decision-making power for health and reproductive decisions. Even women living in nuclear families may face inability to make independent health decisions due to patriarchal attitudes of husband or influence from in-laws. Though many argue that education helps girls and women to make better health decisions, the household support and permission are the final determinant in independent health decisions for women. Studies also highlight that when women own fewer assets, they are allocated less bargaining power in the homes of their husband's and in-laws (Senarath and Gunawardena 2009).

Communication with Family

Decision-making is strongly associated with the type of communication that women have with their parents, husbands, and in-laws. We commonly get confused with the time spent by women in the house and mistake it for high communication with family. In South Asian families, it is not considered culturally acceptable for women to talk about their health, and communication with decision-making family members is limited to discussions about house maintenance and domestic work. A woman may actually spend very few hours with the decision-making family members, and those hours may predominantly be spent eating meals or watching TV. Conversation and discussion usually center around male family members, children, elderly, and household purchases. Many South Asian women can talk to their husbands about community issues, political events, cricket, and matters related to their children, but they cannot talk to them about finances and their health needs (Sathar et al. 2000).

Multiple Births

Possibly the most critical area where South Asian women are prevented by family from making independent health decisions is their choice for reproduction and rights to birth spacing (Howarth and Walker 2011). Pervasive son preference and the social honor associated with the number of sons born in a family in South Asia have major health repercussions on women, both physical and mental. Despite increase in availability and awareness of family planning (Najafi-Sharjabad et al. 2013), many women of South Asia still prefer to have more than two children or to keep having children. In many cases when measuring health decision-making, it is difficult to ascertain whether it is the men or women in the family that sustain pressure on reproduction for the male child. Women may make decisions to assume health risk in persisting with reproduction in order to gain social status with in-laws and in a joint family arrangement and also to secure their conjugal bond with their husband. Ironically, it is also other women, like the mother, mother-in-law, or sister-in-law, who sustain reproductive pressures on other women, thus weakening the gender-based solidarity needed for changing regressive cultural norms influencing women's health. Many women have to opt for clandestine and unsafe abortions and are deprived of postabortion care because of the sustained social pressure for large families and resistance to family planning (Ganatra and Johnston 2002).

It is also common in South Asian families to build pressure for multiple children with the justification that it is important for children to have multiple siblings for their security and support in the future, especially when parents are no longer alive. Having more children or adding to the family-tree branches is also seen as a means of securing and cementing the continuation of the family name and future generations. The South Asian sociocultural ethics supporting the importance of family lineage and large families is more powerful and pervasive than in any other country of the world (Das Gupta et al. 2003; Sathar et al. 2015), and this ethic is more pervasive than prioritizing women's health. The cultural belief is that if a mother dies, she gains heaven and is considered a martyr; thus, she is not encouraged to have fewer children for her health and well-being and instead is encouraged to try for more children until she remains fertile (Roth-Johnson 2018). South Asian families are known to very quickly replace wives or encourage men to remarry in cases of infertility (Thobejane and Flora 2014), and thus, some women may choose to keep reproducing at the cost of their health in order not to be replaced.

Family and Daughters

Maternal health is a grave issue which must be central to policy development because it does not just affect mothers, but the entire family, and especially daughters. The future well-being of families is seriously compromised when mothers' health is compromised and they are unable to contribute to child well-being and nurture, family cohesion and stability, and economic capacity and productivity at national level (Black and Surkan 2015). It is also possible that cycles of adversity can plague children, especially daughters, when their mother is incapacitated, with children having to physically substitute for the duties performed by the mother and having to emotionally deal with the illness of the mother or the loss of mother in the event of mortality (Heath and Tan 2018).

Daughters of South Asia who lose their mothers are commonly forced to assume care roles of cooking, cleaning, and babysitting younger siblings (Khan and Lyon 2015). Daughters may also become more vulnerable to child or early marriage and other forms of abuse, when the mother is not there to protect them (Solotaroff and Pande 2014). As remarriage is common of both widowed men and men with ailing wives in South Asia, children may also have to deal with the problems caused by reconstituted families and neglect and abuse from step mother and other step relations like step brothers and step uncles. This is of grave concern as rape in the home from family members South Asia are known to be high, due to the home being considered a private domain and the social welfare department being inefficient in monitoring home-based abuse.

Child Marriage

Child marriage is prevalent in South Asia, and one of the cultural reasons sustaining the practice is the belief that it is easier to control and manipulate younger girls for a lifetime of domestic service for husband and in-laws (Khanna et al. 2013). The priority of husbands and in-laws is not cultivation of decision-making and autonomy in young girls, but rather robbing them of these qualities. Thus, many South Asian women as child brides are deprived of decision-making for health at marriage, and between domestic drudgery and reproduction, they do not have the time or opportunity to become aware of health needs or assume their rights for health. As children, women are more easily conditioned to believe that as new wives, their status will be elevated through greater reproduction rates and producing multiple children. Similarly, men not only prove their sexual potency through reproduction, but their control of their wives' fertility and health is a cultural symbol of their retained masculinity and honor. Wives who are autonomous and independent become a mark of disrespect for husbands and in-laws. Statistics however confirm that the more times a woman is pregnant and the less she is able to control reproduction and child spacing, the more likely she is to risk her health and also risk her life (Odekunle 2016). Overall, many have concluded that it is the family value system in South Asia that is contributing to female feticide, skewed sex ratios, and gender gap (Abrejo et al. 2009; Amartya 2003). In addition, the skewed gender ratios are not assisted by families who prefer not to try for daughters if the first two children born are sons.

4.3.2 Health Education and Health Behavior

Literacy

With regard to a significant majority of uneducated and semiliterate girls of South Asia, it is evident that they have not received health literacy or awareness from their secondary socializing agents in an academic setting. With regard to women who are attending educational institutes and have not dropped out from the school system, evidence suggests that there is very little health literacy included in the curriculum across South Asia (Abdullah and Zakar 2019). There is also the problem of the hidden curriculum, which teaches girls that health must not be discussed and is an area that is the responsibility of the heads of the household and family. Educating women about health decision-making and how this is not just a right, but that it also preserves the dignity and privacy of women has not been considered. Additionally, the integration of health monitoring in schools, such as immunization, eye and dental checks, counseling, and monitoring for violence and abuse, is nonexistent (Narayanan et al. 2012). This in itself conditions all the genders to believe that health is not a priority and is a personal matter to be dealt with through the rules and norms of the family.

Decisions related to self-health for many South Asian women can also be compared to accepted norms for decisions about sexuality (Cuneo 2018). Both health and sexuality are neither taught nor discussed in the family or the education sector and are not considered culturally acceptable for women to control independently. When self-health is discussed or debated, it is exclusively associated with reproductive health, and in a conservative and patriarchal culture like South Asia, reproductive health is likened to sexuality. Invariably, it is believed that a woman who can control her reproductive health will be licensed to control not just her family size, social order, and traditional norms but also her marital rights and conjugal rights, and this is resisted by united patriarchal forces of the region. Foreign textbooks used in private schools are reprinted without the chapter of "sexuality," in order to suppress any growth or development in this area or assumption of rights.

Health Behavior

Beliefs in South Asia place immense pressure on women for their reproduction role being a natural process and not requiring medical health support or services (Odekunle 2016). Women who require health services for reproduction are not just considered weak and unwomanly, but are also considered plagued by either the burden of their own evils or the victims of the evil eye. This is why many women receive family assistance and cultural support to keep their pregnancies secret and to undertake rituals to ward off evils before conception and delivery. Though the use of traditional and community birth attendants was considered normal in the past, there is still pressure to utilize the community midwife as it is considered as an achievement and a symbol of the dignity and piety of South Asian women in contemporary times. As many women do not have knowledge about the required concoctions, rituals, or midwifery secrets required for a safe delivery, they hand over their decision-making power for health to family and community members with traditional knowledge. It must be remembered that pregnant women are governed by strong emotions and the desperation for a safe delivery with a healthy baby. An emotional woman will always trust her family before "outsiders" in a time when her own and her child's life is at risk. Religious leaders and authoritarians of the community also place a lot of pressure on women to forsake their rights for health decision-making, by using fallacious religious interpretations.

The decisions for continuum of care are not adequate, with many South Asian women preferring to turn to prayer and traditional healing after their recovery through biomedicine (Singh et al. 2016). Women may have been forced to seek biomedical healthcare assistance when in dire need, but they are not known to sustain checkups for health maintenance. There is no concept of eye, dental, and gynecological checkups. Routine self-monitoring of breast and pap smears are considered nonconservative and even perceived as having negative attitudes and not remaining positive. There is family and community pressure to rely on prayer and piety to ward off ill health. In fact, women's health issues are mostly associated with bad character and evilness such as those related to the breast or gynecological areas. This is because social stigmas are powerful and prevalent, placing punitive blame generally on women who fall sick and most especially on women who get breast or ovarian cancer, gynecological problems, or fertility issues (Bedi and Devins 2016). Women from the region also suffer from the stigma of menstruation, with restrictions imposed on menstruating women from: (i) going near male relatives and even young boys, (ii) going near cows, (iii) taking a bath in a pond or lake, and (iv) physical activities like sports and dance (Abrar Aowsaf 2018). At least 40% of school girls surveyed in the National Hygiene Baseline Survey in Bangladesh reported missing school during menstruation (Alam et al. 2017). The stigma leads to less literacy and knowledge about menstrual health and also prevents women and girls from seeking help from practitioners about menstrual problems.

4.3.3 Nature of Employment

Unemployment and Type of Employment

It has generally been assumed that when a woman starts earning an independent income, she will have more decision-making power for her own health needs and for her children. However, this is not always true for South Asian women. There is a complex web of outcomes, with poorer and unskilled working women handing over both their income and their decision-making rights to their husbands (Rhodes et al. 2016). Many upper-class working women in South Asia may also be unable to make decisions for their health autonomously due to cultural norms and social conditioning. Poor women with higher geographical mobility, due to work in the neighborhood or on agricultural land, may have greater decision-making rights for self-health; many would have access problems due to nonavailability of public health services or limited finances for private health services. Nonworking women from the upper-middle-class and rich strata of society may have very little decision-making power or mobility due to conservative and feudal family backgrounds. With regard to the nonworking bracket of women, those who are poor do not have the knowledge, awareness, or finances for health decision-making.

Normally, we associate gender power and autonomous decision-making of women with demographic characteristics of independent income, access to education, and media engagement. However, South Asian cultural norms and social traditions are so powerful that in many cases, they defeat conventional generalizations found in international literature. Working women with independent income and those with media exposure have more awareness for their health needs, but still do not take independent decisions for health, due to excessive need to belong and be culturally accepted. Though broadcast media can play an effective role in women's empowerment for health awareness and rights, there is research to prove that firstly, media is not being used to promote women's health awareness and, secondly, most South Asian women are watching programs on TV that have very little to do with real-life issues and instead are watching serial dramas that sustain regressive custom against women (Linnaeus University 2017). Additionally, exposure to TV does not mean that culturally, women can assume rights for decision-making, as access to TV rarely has an impact on the conservative climate in South Asia related to autonomy in decision-making for women.

4.3.4 Violence and Safety

Low Reportage Culture

There is very low reportage of experiences of domestic violence and workplace violence in South Asia, due to fears of revenge, social shaming, and family dishonor (Mehta 2004). The fact that accountability and swift justice against perpetrators of violence do not work in favor of women is also a strong incentive not to report. Consequently, seeking of health services after experiences of violence is also dismal. Of all the factors that are discussed sustaining domestic violence and workplace violence against women, such as poverty, childlessness, son preference, dowry demands, lower class, and substance abuse, the least discussed is the acceptance of the woman herself. We are arguing that there is a relationship between acceptance of violence and honor codes for disclosing violence, even to healthcare practitioners, thus contributing to low health-seeking behavior in women. Women who are not reporting violence have greater health risks including conception problems, safe delivery of child, survival of child, and life expectancy of woman herself (Acharya et al. 2010).

Ethnicity and Caste

Ethnicity and caste of South Asian women are powerful predictors for decision-making in health. Women who belong to lower caste or are from minority ethnicities have less decision-making power not only within their households but also within the community (Karkee 2012). Women who do have decision-making power are influenced by attitudes of discrimination and prejudice by practitioners and the community. Their alternatives then become opting for self-help, alternative therapy, or traditional local healers from their own caste or ethnicity. Governments and development agents like NGOs often ignore the health needs of marginalized and lower-status minority women, excluding them from program benefits and cash transfers, like the Kammi women of Pakistan (Mumtaz and Mumtaz 2012; Mumtaz et al. 2014). This exclusion is due to structural discrimination prevalent in society but also in order to avoid backlash from majorities, stakeholder, and fund allocators.

Security and Honor Codes

In South Asian countries, regional conflict and security issues have sustained cultural preferences to restrict women's movement and autonomous decision-making, which also affect health access and health behavior (Jamal 2016). Many fathers and husbands prefer that their women manage their health needs within the house and community as it is safer. Additionally, elaborated honor codes enforce the maintenance of the privacy and confidentiality of women's matters and health. Permission is not granted to women in South Asia for independent decision-making to maintain traditions; thus preventing access to health-seeking behavior. In many ways, sustaining women's health decision-making in the hands of the family is seen as a means to preserve the honor, religion, and culture of South Asian societies.

4.3.5 Quality of Healthcare Services and Traditional Healers

Healthcare Practitioner Quality

Decisions for healthcare are also influenced by perceived acceptance and treatment by practitioners in the hospital settings (Zaidi et al. 2017). Problems with practitioners have been a disincentive for South Asian women to seek health services, including issues of lack of informed consent, concealing or not sharing information, preventing decision-making and partnership of patient, cultural incompetency, and even abuse and violence. The organizational climate of clinic and hospitals, especially the public sector, in South Asia is known to be unsafe and discriminatory with perpetrators not just limited to practitioners but also attendants and visitors. Cases of rape and assault are not uncommon (Jafree 2018). Bad experiences with practitioners or having heard about the experiences of others may prompt many women to opt for local healers or delay seeking treatment. Additionally, communities with limited healthcare options and dominant male practitioners or male attendants can become a big disincentive for South Asian women to visit and access.

Trust and confidence in medical practitioners and the health workforce are an essential component driving health decisions. When families are making the decisions for health of woman, their conservative orientations would lean toward traditional healthcare solutions and traditional healers (Amin et al. 2015; Khaliq et al. 2019). Women themselves may feel more comfortable and secure in accessing traditional solutions for health due to fear of biomedical interventions, unnecessary surgical interventions, and permanent damage to reproductive health. Many South Asian women have greater respect and trust in their traditional healers because of association, kinship, or likeness in ethnicity or religion. Also, the ratios of healthcare practitioners to population are far less, compared to availability and convenience of untrained healers in the community. Thus, rational and practical reasons for opting for community healers are also a consideration for South Asian women. There has been great effort in South Asia to train community providers to give safe services for women (van Weel et al. 2016). However, even in the event of community healers having a license or receiving skilled training, lack of provision of surgical and clinical facilities and other medical equipment may contribute to mortality or adverse health risks in women (Jafree et al. 2018). This is why those with independent health decision-making also prefer traditional healthcare services due to cultural norms, access, cost, and fears of unnecessary and harmful biomedical intervention.

4.3.6 Resource Shortages

Decisions for uptake at health centers are not just influenced by resources and practitioners but also by the availability of energy supply. As majority of women in South Asia reside in rural areas, the quality of energy supply at primary health centers is not the best (Thapa 2005). Decisions for health access from a health center are influenced by multiple structural factors like women's distance and the availability and affordability of transport and the perceived safety in travel to health center (Babinard and Roberts 2006). Culturally, women may be abused and shamed for visiting a health center that is known in the community not to be functional or have sufficient resources. Similarly, women who want to travel to health centers without male relatives may face permission issues and cultural barriers (Banu 2016). It has been evidenced that South Asian women are also not allowed to attain health services due to family fears that they will adopt family planning or opt for covert abortions (Farid et al. 2013; Grimes et al. 2006). In this way, many women prefer to take their husband or a member of their in-laws as a witness for what they were actually seeking medical help for.

Health Surveillance

Women of South Asia are more affected by the panoptic surveillance and the fears of information sharing than any other group of women in the world (World Health Organization 2005). Though we live in the age of big data and demographic surveillance, South Asian families may still be reluctant to share data related to their women, as this is culturally considered a private domain. One of the fears of families in visiting primary health centers is that they might record information, which can be retrieved by community members. Demographic data particularly facts like age of women, house address, contact numbers, engagement with media, her health history, and abortion history are all areas that families and women themselves prefer not to share or have recorded. Women themselves are reluctant to share their data with health centers as they are suspicious of what may be done with this data and the possibility of compromising their safety and status in society and the community. It is also not unknown for traditional communities in South Asia to consider Western health practices and treatment a means of surveillance and harm to local population, like in the case of assuming that polio vaccines affect fertility (Andrade and Hussain 2018).

Community Providers

Causes of maternal deaths are empirically also related to lack of institutional deliveries, which is definitely a case of limited access but also a result of lack of permission and regressive beliefs (El-Saharty et al. 2016). Though skilled birth attendants are still critically short in ratio to population and there are issues of skilled attendants not increasing in ratio compared to population rates, one of the main barriers remains cultural rejection of trained community providers. Research confirms that community healthcare workers are scarce in Pakistan, Bangladesh, and India and that even when available, they are not being used in rural areas due to cultural reasons (Islam et al. 2014). Decisions for taking health services from trained community providers are also influenced by the belief that nontraditional health solutions and counsel are being provided. Many women are not given permission or are abused for taking assistance from trained community providers. This community resistance and patriarchal rejection is the reason why many community workers suffer from abuse and violence and are no longer considered part of the community after they assume Western biomedical training (Jafree 2018). Many families and men refuse to let their women seek services from community providers, and many women themselves refuse to seek help from trained community providers in order to retain their identity as the obliging and conservative woman of the house.

Most of the community workers that are recruited are young and below the age of 35 years, and many have not had children (Family Health Division Ministry of Health 2008). It is easier to train younger women and rely on their energy for work in the community, with the expectation that they will serve the community for a longer period of years. However, again in conservative South Asian climates, there is a tradition for trusting older women who are believed to have more experience and also women who have had more children themselves. In addition, the elder and experienced community midwife who has delivered more than a hundred children in the village will always be more trusted than the younger community worker who has received training for a few weeks and is getting money from the government (Hafeez et al. 2011). The community midwife also has more emotional connections and may accept cash or kind, which for poorer and traditional people provides a more tangible reasoning for why she is helping them, compared to the government worker.

4.4 Conclusion

To meet the Sustainable Development Goals (SDG) for maternal and child health, gender equality, health access for all, and poverty reduction (Jha et al. 2016), it is critical that South Asian governments take responsibility for the financial support of women's health. We have found in the chapter, through chi-square results, some of the salient demographic and social areas that need assistance for independent health decision-making: (i) younger and older women between the ages of 15 and 49 years, (ii) illiterate and literate women, (iii) rural women, (iv) poor women, (v) women with less than four children, (vi) women who are not working, (vii) women who are not paid in cash, (viii) women who do not watch TV, (ix) women who do not have or have not seen an immunization card of their child, and (x) women who do not believe that beating is justified.

Massive mobilization is needed for poverty alleviation of women in South Asia. Feminization of poverty can become embedded in social structures and become an accepted part of the socioeconomic culture. Removing women from cyclical poverty requires systematic and well-planned policies for cash transfers and loan provision. Keeping women out of poverty will require more than financial injections, such as simultaneous policies promoting enrollment in the education sector and formal sector work participation. Legal accountability is needed for minimum wage allowances, along with protection and employment benefits for maternity, sickness, and retirement. Population growth for all three countries is expected to double within the next few decades with growth rates in Pakistan even more alarming than other countries (D'Ensemble 2019). This suggests more problems related to shortages for health resources, health services, and health budgets, with women and the girl child expected to suffer more than the men. Population growth will also have a greater effect on food shortages, water scarcity, and undernutrition in women and girls. In addition, reproductive pressures and multiple births are known to have a correlation with health problems and even mortality in women. We have known for many years that women of South Asia are deprived of universal health coverage (Scammell et al. 2016). However, the rural woman is more vulnerable to health challenges of access, affordability, and permission. As majority of women of South Asia are residing in rural areas, there is need for concentrated efforts for rural healthcare services for maternal health need, more planning, budget allocation, resources, research, and accountability for reproductive health.

In South Asia, female education has been low, and this has been touted as one of the reasons for inability to attain targets for women's health improvements (Bhutta and Black 2013). There is a critical role for health literacy and health awareness campaigns across the region, encompassing not just women, but male members of the family. South Asian governments have concentrated on introducing awareness and programs for family planning, without attempting to change social factors which compel the demand for large families, namely, poverty, culture, and religious interpretation. The role of religious leader, tribal leaders, elders in the community, and male family members is essential in changing religious and traditional norms. Educational curricula and health literacy must include awareness for health needs of women and link it to the development of nation and future of our children. Health literacy must also include education of young boys about the autonomy of women's health decision-making in context to privacy and inability of women to discuss all matters related to their health with men and in-laws. With the stress on religious education for many South Asian women, religious fallacies and illegitimate religious scholars have not provided a means for optimal health access and self-care (Inman 2006).

Many South Asian interventions have concentrated on improving health outcomes like increasing institutional access for deliveries and training skilled attendants from outside the community (van Weel et al. 2016). However, these interventions have not been as successful as expected due to cultural barriers. Though community enablers have been labeled as the best means to alter and reform community norms in favor of women's health, community enablers are not widely prevalent, consistent, or accepted across the South Asian region. Some urban zones and small citizenship programs are not sufficient to transform cultural traditions toward enabling women to make autonomous decisions for health (Kidney et al. 2009). In Bangladesh, cash transfers were provided to poor parents with strict conditions that they must send their daughter to school. However, increase in enrollment and cash transfers have not secured changed community norms for allowing independent decision-making for women. Last, we must also consider what the effect of inability to control health decision-making might have on women both emotionally and physically (Shooshtari et al. 2018). There is thus simultaneous need for incorporation of mental health support for women of South Asia robbed for years of self-determination.

To assume that South Asian women are homogeneous and one health policy can reform the lives of all the women collectively would be too simplistic. Ultimately, health decisions for autonomous health decision-making in South Asian women are influenced by social constructions and cultural interpretations for: (i) traditions and historical legacies, (ii) religious beliefs, and (iii) family honor. If there is a magic bullet, it would have to be cultural reform for women's acceptability in making health decisions autonomously. There is thus need for micro community-level interventions of different natures and degrees to benefit the heterogeneous populations controlled by culture and traditions. Isolated male partner interventions for birth spacing and maternal health are not enough. A more macro approach of father-brother-husband interventions with male community notables is also needed to understand the importance of women's health literacy and health decision-making through the age course and its impact on family and child well-being.

References

Abdullah, M., & Zakar, R. (2019). Health literacy in South Asia: Clarifying the connections between health literacy and wellbeing in Pakistan. *Health, 34*(2), 575–589.

Abrar Aowsaf, S. M. (2018). World Menstrual Hygiene Day: Menstruation taboos pose major health risks for Bangladeshi women. *Dhaka Tribune.* Retrieved from https://www.dhakatribune.com/opinion/special/2018/05/28/world-menstrual-hygiene-day-menstruation-taboos-pose-major-health-risks-for-bangladeshi-women

Abrejo, F. G., Shaikh, B. T., & Rizvi, N. (2009). 'And they kill me, only because I am a girl' ... a review of sex-selective abortions in South Asia. *The European Journal of Contraception Reproductive Health Care, 14*(1), 10–16.

Acharya, D. R., Bell, J. S., Simkhada, P., Van Teijlingen, E. R., & Regmi, P. R. (2010). Women's autonomy in household decision-making: A demographic study in Nepal. *Reproductive Health, 7*(1), 15.

Akseer, N., Kamali, M., Arifeen, S. E., Malik, A., Bhatti, Z., Thacker, N., et al. (2017). Progress in maternal and child health: How has South Asia fared? *BMJ, 357*, j1608.

Alam, M., Halder, A., & Horng, L. (2017). *Bangladesh national hygiene baseline survey preliminary report.* Dhaka: International Centre for Diarrheal Diseases Research.

Allendorf, K. (2017). Like her own: Ideals and experiences of the mother-in-law/daughter-in-law relationship. *Journal of Family Issues, 38*(15), 2102–2127.

Amartya, S. (2003). *Missing women – Revisited.* British Medical Journal Publishing Group.

Amin, F., Islam, N., & Gilani, A. (2015). Traditional and complementary/alternative medicine use in a south-Asian population. *Asian Pacific Journal of Health Sciences, 2*, 36–42.

Andrade, G. E., & Hussain, A. (2018). Polio in Pakistan: Political, sociological, and epidemiological factors. *Cureus, 10*(10).

Babinard, J., & Roberts, P. (2006). *Maternal and child mortality development goals: What can the transport sector do?* The International Bank for Reconstruction and Development/The World

Bank, https://openknowledge.worldbank.org/bitstream/handle/10986/17413/373660tp120Mat1development01PUBLIC1.pdf?sequence=1&isAllowed=y

Banu, A. (2016). *Human development, disparity and vulnerability: Women in South Asia*. Background paper for Human Development Report.

Bedi, M., & Devins, G. M. (2016). Cultural considerations for South Asian women with breast cancer. *Journal of Cancer Survivorship, 10*(1), 31–50.

Bhutta, Z. A., & Black, R. E. (2013). Global maternal, newborn, and child health—So near and yet so far. *New England Journal of Medicine, 369*(23), 2226–2235.

Black, M. M., & Surkan, P. J. (2015). Child development and maternal wellbeing: Family perspectives for low-income and middle-income countries. *The Lancet Global Health, 3*(8), e426–e427.

Cuneo, D. (2018). Sociocultural constructions of sexuality in South Asia. Kervan. *International Journal of Afro-Asiatic Studies* (21).

D'Ensemble, V. U. E. (2019). *World population prospects 2019: Highlights*. United Nations.

Das Gupta, M., Zhenghua, J., Bohua, L., Zhenming, X., Chung, W., & Hwa-Ok, B. (2003). Why is son preference so persistent in East and South Asia? A cross-country study of China, India and the Republic of Korea. *The Journal of Development Studies, 40*(2), 153–187.

Desai, S., & Johnson, K. (2005). *Women's decision making and child health: familial and social hierarchies*. In A focus on gender: Collected papers on gender using DHS data (Vol. 2005, pp. 55–68). ORC Macro Calverton, MD.

El-Saharty, S., Chowdhury, S., Ohno, N., & Sarker, I. (2016). *Improving maternal and reproductive health in South Asia: Drivers and enablers*. Washington, DC: The World Bank.

Family Health Division Ministry of Health, Nepal. (2008). *An analytical report on national survey of female community health volunteers of Nepal*. Female Community Health Volunteers Report, Retrieved from https://dhsprogram.com/pubs/pdf/FR181/FCHV_Nepal2007.pdf.

Farid, H., Siddique, S. M., Bachmann, G., Janevic, T., & Pichika, A. (2013). Practice of and attitudes towards family planning among South Asian American immigrants. *Journal of Contraception, 88*(4), 518–522.

Ganatra, B., & Johnston, H. B. (2002). Reducing abortion-related mortality in South Asia: A review of constraints and a road map for change. *Journal of the American Medical Women's Association, 57*(3), 159–164.

Godha, D., Hotchkiss, D. R., & Gage, A. J. (2013). Association between child marriage and reproductive health outcomes and service utilization: A multi-country study from South Asia. *Journal of Adolescent Health, 52*(5), 552–558.

Grimes, D. A., Benson, J., Singh, S., Romero, M., Ganatra, B., Okonofua, F. E., & Shah, I. H. (2006). Unsafe abortion: The preventable pandemic. *The lancet, 368*(9550), 1908–1919.

Hafeez, A., Mohamud, B. K., Shiekh, M. R., Shah, S. A. I., & Jooma, R. (2011). Lady health workers programme in Pakistan: Challenges, achievements and the way forward. *JPMA: Journal of the Pakistan Medical Association, 61*(3), 210.

Heath, R., & Tan, X. (2018). Worth fighting for: Daughters improve their mothers' autonomy in South Asia. *Journal of Development Economics, 135*, 255–271.

Howarth, L., & Walker, J. (2011). The role of family planning in South Asia. *BJOG: an international journal of obstetrics gynaecology, 118*, 31–35.

Inman, A. G. (2006). South Asian women: Identities and conflicts. *Cultural Diversity and Ethnic Minority Psychology, 12*(2), 306.

Islam, N., Islam, M. T., & Yoshimura, Y. (2014). Practices and determinants of delivery by skilled birth attendants in Bangladesh. *Reproductive Health, 11*(1), 86.

Jafree, S. R. (2018). *Women, healthcare, and violence in Pakistan*. Karachi: Oxford University Press.

Jafree, S. R., Zakar, R., Mustafa, M., & Fischer, F. (2018). Mothers employed in paid work and their predictors for home delivery in Pakistan. *BMC Pregnancy Childbirth, 18*(1), 316.

Jamal, A. (2016). Why he Won't send his daughter to school—Barriers to girls' education in Northwest Pakistan: A qualitative Delphi study of Pashtun men. *SAGE Open, 6*(3).

Jejeebhoy, S. J., & Sathar, Z. A. (2001). Women's autonomy in India and Pakistan: The influence of religion and region. *Population and Development Review, 27*(4), 687–712.

Jha, A., Kickbusch, I., Taylor, P., & Abbasi, K. (2016). Accelerating achievement of the sustainable development goals. *British Medical Journal, 352*, i409.

Karkee, R. (2012). How did Nepal reduce the maternal mortality? A result from analysing the determinants of maternal mortality. *Journal of the Nepal Medical Association, 52*(186).

Khaliq, I. H., Mahmood, H. Z., Sarfraz, M. D., Gondal, K. M., & Zaman, S. (2019). Pathways to care for patients in Pakistan experiencing signs or symptoms of breast cancer. *The Breast, 46*, 40–47.

Khan, S. R., & Lyon, S. (2015). *Measuring children's work in South Asia: Perspectives from national household surveys*. New Delhi: ILO.

Khanna, T., Verma, R., & Weiss, E. (2013). *Child marriage in South Asia: Realities responses and the way forward*. New Delhi: International Centre for Research.

Kidney, E., Winter, H. R., Khan, K. S., Gülmezoglu, A. M., Meads, C. A., Deeks, J. J., & MacArthur, C. (2009). Systematic review of effect of community-level interventions to reduce maternal mortality. *BMC Pregnancy and Childbirth, 9*(1), 2.

Lee, C. K., & Beatty, S. E. (2002). Family structure and influence in family decision making. *Journal of Consumer Marketing, 19*(1), 24–41.

Leopold, T. A., Ratcheva, V., & Zahidi, S. (2016). *The global gender gap report 2016*. Paper presented at the World Economic Forum.

Linnaeus University. (2017). *A changing Asian media assessing challenges and opportunities for evolving media in South and SouthEast Asia* (International Media Support and FOJO Media Institute Report).

Marphatia, A. A., Ambale, G. S., & Reid, A. M. (2017). Women's marriage age matters for public health: A review of the broader health and social implications in South Asia. *Frontiers in Public Health, 5*, 269.

Mehta, M. (2004). *Towards ending violence against women in South Asia*. Oxfam International.

Mumtaz, K., & Mumtaz, S. (2012). Women's participation in the Punjab peasant movement: From community rights to women's rights? Political conflict and women in South Asia'. *South Asia Journal, 35*, 138–150.

Mumtaz, Z., & Salway, S. (2009). Understanding gendered influences on women's reproductive health in Pakistan: Moving beyond the autonomy paradigm. *Social Science Medicine, 68*(7), 1349–1356.

Mumtaz, Z., Salway, S., Bhatti, A., Shanner, L., Zaman, S., Laing, L., & Ellison, G. T. (2014). Improving maternal health in Pakistan: Toward a deeper understanding of the social determinants of poor women's access to maternal health services. *American Journal of Public Health, 104*(S1), S17–S24.

Najafi-Sharjabad, F., Yahya, S. Z. S., Hejar Abdul Rahman, M. H., & Manaf, R. A. (2013). Barriers of modern contraceptive practices among Asian women: A mini literature review. *Global Journal of health science, 5*(5), 181.

Narayanan, R., van Norden, H., Gosling, L., & Patkar, A. (2012). Equity and inclusion in sanitation and hygiene in South Asia: A regional synthesis. *IDS Bulletin, 43*(2), 101–111.

Odekunle, F. F. (2016). Maternal mortality burden: The influence of sociocultural factors. *International Journal of Health Sciences and Research, 6*(12), 316–324.

Rhodes, F., Burnley, J., Dolores, M., Kyriacou, J., Wilshaw, R., Ukhova, D., … & Talpur, M. . (2016). *Underpaid and Undervalued: How inequality defines women's work in Asia* (Oxfam report).

Roth-Johnson, D. (2018). Muslim mothering: Global histories, theories, and practices. *Journal of the Motherhood Initiative for Research Community Involvement, 9*(1).

Sathar, Z. A., & Kazi, S. (2000). Women's autonomy in the context of rural Pakistan. *The Pakistan Development Review*, 89–110.

Sathar, Z. A., Kazi, S., & Mahmood, A. (2000). Pakistani couples: Different productive and reproductive realities?[with comments]. *The Pakistan Development Review*, 891–912.

Sathar, Z. A., Rashida, G., Hussain, S., & Hassan, A. (2015). *Evidence of son preference and resulting demographic and health outcomes in Pakistan*. Islamabad: Population Council.
Scammell, K., Noble, D. J., Rasanathan, K., O'Connell, T., Ahmed, A. S., Begkoyian, G., et al. (2016). A landscape analysis of universal health coverage for mothers and children in South Asia. *BMJ Global Health, 1*(1).
Senarath, U., & Gunawardena, N. S. (2009). Women's autonomy in decision making for health care in South Asia. *Asia Pacific Journal of Public Health, 21*(2), 137–143.
Sheikh, S. M., & Loney, T. (2018). Is educating girls the best Investment for South Asia? Association between female education and fertility choices in South Asia: A systematic review of the literature. *Frontiers in Public Health, 6*, 172.
Shooshtari, S., Abedi, M. R., Bahrami, M., & Samouei, R. (2018). Empowerment of women and mental health improvement with a preventive approach. *Journal of Education and Health Promotion, 7*.
Singh, K., Story, W. T., & Moran, A. C. (2016). Assessing the continuum of care pathway for maternal health in South Asia and sub-Saharan Africa. *Maternal and Child Health Journal, 20*(2), 281–289.
Solotaroff, J. L., & Pande, R. P. (2014). *Violence against women and girls: Lessons from South Asia*. Washington, DC: The World Bank.
Thapa, G. (2005). Rural poverty reduction strategy for South Asia. In: *Economic Growth, Economic Performance and Welfare in South Asia* (pp. 384–401). Springer.
Thobejane, T. D., & Flora, T. (2014). An exploration of polygamous marriages: A worldview. *Mediterranean Journal of Social Sciences, 5*(27 P2), 1058.
van Weel, C., Kassai, R., Qidwai, W., Kumar, R., Bala, K., Gupta, P. P., et al. (2016). Primary healthcare policy implementation in South Asia. *BMJ Global Health, 1*(2), e000057.
World Health Organization. (2005). *Evaluating the costs and benefits of national surveillance and response systems: methodologies and options*. Retrieved from.
Wusu, O., & Isiugo-Abanihe, U. C. (2003). Family structure and reproductive health decision making among the Ogu of southwestern Nigeria: A qualitative study. *African Population Studies, 18*(2).
Zaidi, S., Saligram, P., Ahmed, S., Sonderp, E., & Sheikh, K. (2017). Expanding access to healthcare in South Asia. *British Medical Journal, 357*, j1645.

Chapter 5
Poverty, Health Coverage, and Credit Opportunities for South Asian Women

Fionnuala Gormley and Sara Rizvi Jafree

5.1 Introduction

We begin this chapter by considering different definitions of poverty and the term feminization of poverty. Townsend (2006) outlines three conceptions of poverty that have evolved since the 1880s, based principally on the ideas of: (i) subsistence, (ii) basic needs, and (iii) relative deprivation. The subsistence idea as a poverty measure was devised by nutritionists in England during the Victorian period. Families whose income after rent was insufficient to ensure proper nutrition were treated as being in poverty. The "basic needs" approach was introduced by the International Labour Organization's World Employment Conference in 1976 (Dharam 1999). The basic needs of a family included a minimum level of consumption of food including water, shelter, and clothing. Many modern lists now also include the minimum level of consumption of additional "basic needs" of sanitation, education, healthcare, and Internet. Within rural areas, basic needs also include land, agricultural tools, and access to farming.

In the late twentieth century, a third formulation known as relative poverty was developed based on relative deprivation. People falling under the category of relative poverty are not living in total poverty, but they are not enjoying the same standard of life as everyone else within their country. The term ultra-poor originates from Lipton (1986). It is defined as "a group of people who eat below 80% of their energy requirements despite spending at least 80% of income on food." The concept of "feminization of poverty" gained popularity in the 1990s following its usage within United Nations reports (United Nations 2000). Feminization of poverty

F. Gormley (✉)
Global Market Risk Management Department, London, UK

S. R. Jafree
Department of Sociology, Forman Christian College University, Lahore, Pakistan

S. R. Jafree (ed.), *The Sociology of South Asian Women's Health*,
https://doi.org/10.1007/978-3-030-50204-1_5

Table 5.1 Population and labor force participation rates for women and men in South Asian countries[a]

	Bangladesh		India		Pakistan		Sri Lanka	
	Women	Men	Women	Men	Women	Men	Women	Men
Population share 2017[b]								
National	49.6%	50.4%	48.2%	51.8%	48.6%	51.4%	51.9%	48.1%
Labor force participation in 2017[c]								
National	36.4%	80.7%	23.4%	79.1%	21.9%	80.4%	35.8%	75.0%
Rural	38.6%	80.5%	25.7%	80.5%	28.1%	82.3%	36.9%	75.5%
Urban	31.0%	81.2%	17.8%	76.0%	11.7%	77.5%	30.2%	72.6%

[a]Data in this table has been compiled by the authors from secondary data sources
[b]This data has been retrieved from publically available data-sets by STATISTA
[c]This data source has been retrieved from publically available data-sets by International Labor Organization

refers to the phenomenon of a widening gap between women and men who are caught in a cycle of economic scarcity and deprivation. Several factors have been identified as causes of poverty among women. What we will concentrate on in this chapter is the relationship between poverty, employment, and health (life expectancy indicator) of women in South Asia.

Table 5.1 shows us that nearly 50% of the population of Bangladesh, India, and Pakistan are women, at 49.6%, 48.2%, and 48.6% respectively; whereas in Sri Lanka women exceed men at 51.9%. However, women comprise less than 36% of the labor force across all four countries (Bangladesh = 36.4%; India = 23.4%; Pakistan = 21.9%; and Sri Lanka = 35.8%).

Table 5.2 shows that the life expectancy of women in South Asia at 71 years is far below average life expectancy found in other parts of Asia (East Asia = 80; Western Asia = 77; Central Asia = 76; South East Asia = 75). This is primarily because women from South Asia compared to other parts of Asia still face eco-social and political barriers to gender equality (Selvaratnam 1988). Majority of women in South Asia at 50.7% live in poverty, and a significant number of educated women (with education at primary, secondary or tertiary level combined) also live in poverty, at 23.7%. Of further relevance is that even women working in paid employment and those who are self-employed are living in poverty, at 27.0%. The data compels us to ask why large numbers of educated and working women in South Asia also face crippling poverty.

5.2 Determinants of Poverty

The key determinants of poverty for South Asia are cultural and political, and this section will discuss those factors in more detail, including: (i) family composition, (ii) control over resources, (iii) access to education and health, (iv) inequality in social protection, and (v) labor market inequalities.

Table 5.2 Life expectancy and poverty data for South Asia[a]

	Women	Men	*Diff*
Average life expectancy for those born in 2019, in years[b]			
	71	68	*3*
Population living in poverty in2018[c]			
	50.7%	49.3%	*0.01*
Poverty rates by education level in 2018[c]			
No education	20.5%	21.9%	*−0.01*
Primary	14.1%	16.4%	*−0.02*
Secondary	7.9%	9.7%	*−0.02*
Tertiary	1.7%	2.1%	*0.00*
Poverty rates by employment status in 2018[c]			
Paid worker	16.6%	14.0%	*0.03*
Unpaid worker	14.8%	16.5%	*−0.02*
Self-employed	10.4%	11.8%	*−0.01*
Unemployed	7.0%	6.7%	*0.00*
Out of labor force	13.3%	9.5%	*0.04*

[a]Data in this table has been compiled by the authors from secondary data sources
[b]This data has been retrieved from publically available data-sets by STATISTA
[c]This data source has been retrieved from publically available data-sets by World Bank Group

5.2.1 Family Composition

Family composition distinguishes between different types of families, based on dissolution of marital unions, constitution of families without these unions, and higher male mortality. In India, marriage, divorce, succession, maintenance, adoption, guardianship, and child custody continue to be governed by the laws defined by various religious communities. A review of these laws carried out by Cossman and Kapur (2008) identified many laws which discriminated on the basis of gender. An example of these laws is the Hindu Marriage Act of 1956 which does not allow a divorced woman an equal share of property, income, and assets unless the assets are in joint names or were gifts before or at the time of her wedding.

Women's contribution, both direct and indirect, to the acquisition and maintenance of assets during the marital relationship is therefore likely to be unrewarded if the assets were registered in the husband's or his family's name. Such laws increase the economic dependency of women on their family across all social classes and result in socioeconomic inequality. An informal worker survey carried out in Srivastava's research (2013) found that women who were abandoned or whose husbands were missing were at risk of poverty when both the responsibilities of household work and income generation fell on them. Many widows lacked documentation to obtain widow pensions or may be ruled out of pension schemes if their husbands had left them. Other significant challenges include awareness and childcare support. Many women are often unaware of social protection schemes available to them, and widows or abandoned wives with young children often face difficulty in accessing paid work due to the absence of childcare.

5.2.2 Control over Resources

A second factor contributing to poverty relates to gender roles regulating the control over household resources as well as the gendered division of labor and consumption within households. Srivastava (2013) highlighted that the decision for women to marry at a young age in India often arose from cultural practices and was decided by families rather than women themselves. Early marriage resulted in increased family size, poorer health, and dismal living standards for women and their children. According to the National Family Health Survey of India (NFHS) 2015–2016, 31.1% of Indian women have experienced spousal violence during their lives. Das and Mehta (2012) analyzed women who had experienced spousal violence during the 12 months prior to the NFHS-3 survey. They found that women were least likely to experience violence if they had education beyond secondary level and were from the wealthier section of society. A study by Panda and Agarwal (2005) based on a 2001 household survey carried out in Kerala (Thiruvananthapuram district) reported that women who owned land or property were much less likely to experience physical and mental violence. It is expected that land and property ownership increases women's safety because in the face of violence they could leave and still maintain financial security. The Hindu Succession (Amendment) Act of 2005 has removed gender discriminatory provisions regarding property inheritance rights that had been laid out in the Hindu Succession Act of 1956. Under the 2005 amendment, daughters have the same property inheritance rights as sons. However, culture and traditions still compel many parents to leave most of their property to sons as they believe their sons will take care of them in their old age.

A review of Gender and Land Rights Database of United Nations Food and Agricultural Organization (GLRD, UN FAO) shows that worldwide women's ownership of agricultural land is generally very low. In Bangladesh, just 4.8% of agricultural land holdings belonged to women, according to the 2008 Agricultural Census, while in India the figure was 12.8% as recorded in the 2010–2011 Agricultural Census. Women's legal entitlement to property and alimony can leave them disadvantaged within Bangladesh. Under Islamic law, daughters inherit half the property that is given to sons, while daughters of Hindus and Buddhists are not entitled to any inheritance. Davis (2011) conducted 293 interviews in rural Bangladesh to identify how families emerged from poverty. The most frequently cited reasons were: (i) ownership of small businesses, (ii) the acquisition of assets such as land and cattle, and (iii) income from sons and daughters.

The Household Income and Expenditure Survey of Bangladesh, HIES 2010, calculated estimates of headcount rate (HCR) of poverty using the upper poverty line measure. Landless households earned income from sectors outside the agricultural division and recorded lower rates of poverty than households with very small land holdings. The HCR using the upper poverty line was 35.4% for households who did not own land and 45.1% for households with holdings of less than 0.05 acres. Thus, poverty rates of households are observed to decline with land ownership. The HIES 2010 survey estimated that 48% of the population of Bangladesh were earning their living through farming. HIES 2010 also analyzed poverty rates in rural vs. urban areas in Bangladesh in 2005 and 2010. Poverty rates in rural areas were higher than in urban areas. In 2010, instances of poverty using the upper poverty line were 21.3% for urban areas in Bangladesh and 35.2% in rural areas.

5.2.3 Access to Education and Health

A third factor causing feminization of poverty is caused by inequality in access to education and healthcare services. According to the National Family Health Survey of 2015–2016, NFHS-4 of India, the percentage of women in India aged 20–24 years who were married before the age of 18 years was 26.8% at a national level in 2015. Early marriage can result in reduced access to education. Literacy was identified as another important factor in poverty rates in Bangladesh in HIES 2010. In 2010, poverty rates in Bangladesh using the upper poverty line were 19.0% for literates and 42.8% for the illiterates, a gap of 23.8%. Umme and Malik (2012) explored poverty rates in Bangladesh among highly educated women. Their study showed that a higher percentage of educated women are poorer than educated men because a larger proportion are housewives which reduces their opportunity to use their education to earn income, access social security, and engage in social interaction outside of their household. If education is regarded as an investment in income generation, women who have fewer labor market opportunities may be less likely to invest in education, have lower earnings, and be more likely to experience poverty.

Similar findings were observed in a study carried by Siddiqui and Hamid (2009) in Pakistan. The incidence of poverty was found to be higher among households with female heads, especially in rural areas. The authors identified education as the most effective means of poverty reduction and improvements in women's status in Pakistan. Lower literacy rates were observed for girls due to gender discrimination because the return on investment in girl's education was seen as lower than that of boys. The benefits of access to education for women included improvements in mental health, participation in paid work, and opportunities for asset ownership.

5.2.4 Social Protection Inequality

A fourth factor giving rise to poverty for women relates to inequality in social protection floors. The term "social protection floor" is a concept developed by the International Labor Organization (ILO) which is used to describe a minimum set of social rights, facilities, and services that citizens of a nation should have access to (SPF Advisory Group 2011). The purpose of a social protection floor is to prevent and alleviate poverty, vulnerability, and social exclusion through: (i) guarantees of basic income; (ii) security covering pensions for the elderly, the sick, and the disabled; (iii) child benefits; and (iv) income support and services for the unemployed.

It also includes access to essential social services that include water, sanitation, food, housing, healthcare, and education. In countries without a fully functioning social protection floor, it is often women who are the most adversely affected. This is because women have fewer employment opportunities and greater responsibility for the care of children and elderly parents. Lower income potential and informal work have a knock-on impact on financial stability both in terms of savings and preparation for old age in working women. Even today, it is the South Asian mother who will leave the workforce to rear the children as culturally there is little acceptance for paternal assistance.

5.2.5 *Labor Market Inequalities*

Another factor giving rise to poverty for women relates to labor market inequalities. One of the primary economic causes of poverty among Bangladeshi women identified by Holmes et al. (2010) was the differences in the labor participation rate between men and women. Women in Bangladesh have lower participation rates in paid labor than men, although rates have risen in recent years with the development of the garment industry in Bangladesh. However, on average, women are paid less compared to men within the same role and occupy a higher proportion of lower paid roles overall. As men move away from the agricultural sector into higher paying sectors, the participation rate for women in the agricultural sector is increasing, leaving them in a sector which sustains them in poverty and inequality. As we saw in Table 5.1, men's participation in the labor force is far higher than that of women ranging from 38% to 66%. Low labor force participation rates of women in South Asian countries contribute to a gender gap in wages. Empirical evidence suggests that when labor participation rates of women increase, it contributes to economic growth and reduced poverty not just for women but for the whole household, with most benefits reaped by children (Ki-Moon 2010).

5.3 Financial Risks of South Asian Women Working in the Informal Sector

The 2018 World Economic Forum Global Gender Report, WEF 2018, analyzed 149 countries on their progress toward gender parity on a scale from 0 (disparity) to 1 (parity). Specific areas where gender disparity is observed for Bangladesh, India, Sri Lanka, and Pakistan include: (i) financial and political power and (ii) economic participation and opportunity. Much of this inequality is because of high rates of women's unemployment and overrepresentation in the informal sector. The term informal sector is used to specify that segment of the economy, which has absorbed significant numbers of job seekers and unemployed workers outside government regulations and formal systems of labor and social protection. Not only are majority women in South Asia unpaid domestic labor, but the working women of the region are predominantly part of the informal sector. As informal workers, they are known to be home-based workers, thus falling easily through gaps in enumeration as data and statistics on household level are still difficult to measure. In 2008, 70% of South Asian women were engaged in paid work in the agricultural sector (ILO 2010). Own-account workers or contributing family workers are identified as "vulnerable employment" by the International Labor Organization (ILO 2010). The number of females in the labor force is continuously on the rise, and the actual number of women in the informal economy is probably much more than reflected in the available statistics.

A study carried out by the International Labor Organization found that 72% of workers in South Asia were in vulnerable employment. Vulnerable employment rates for women in South Asia are 8% higher than those of men (ILO 2018). Employment in the informal sector ranges between 70% and 90% in Sri Lanka, Pakistan, India, and Bangladesh. The potential to reduce poverty rates in South Asia is undermined by high rates of informal work. Higher rates of informality are observed in certain sectors, in particular, the agriculture sector and nonagricultural sectors including construction, retail trade, accommodation, and food service industries (ILO 2018). According to a World Health Organization publication in 2005, 150 million people suffer financial catastrophe annually, and 100 million people are pushed below the poverty line when compelled to pay for healthcare (WHO 2005). Given the high rate of informal work in South Asia, it is estimated that just one in five women are covered by adequate social security (ILO 2011). Srivastava (2013) identified that women working in the informal sector in India faced occupational health issues. Access to healthcare was often inaccessible leading to delays in workers seeking treatment until serious symptoms occurred. For some women, the formalization of work caused them to lose out on roles which they had previously undertaken in the informal sector, such as health supervision and food preparation for self and children.

The Indian Economy is characterized by a large section of the economy employed within an informal labor market. The National Statistical Commission 2012, reported that over 90 per cent of the workforce and approximately 50% of the national product were accounted for by the informal economy. Two of the most significant labor laws enacted in India to protect and promote the particular interests of women workers are the Maternity Benefit Act, 1961 (MBA 1961), and the subsequent amendment the Maternity Benefit (Amendment) Act 2017 (MBAA 2017). The Maternity Benefit (Amendment) Act 2017 increased the duration of paid maternity leave from 12 weeks to 26 weeks. Pregnant women are also entitled to take up to 8 weeks paid leave of absence prior to their expected date of delivery, with the remaining time to be taken after delivery. The Act also makes childcare facilities mandatory for every workplace employing 50 or more employees with female employees permitted to visit the childcare up to four times per day.

However, there are serious limitations to the maternity policy in India. The cost of maternity benefits is fully paid for by employers. This is in contrast to most other countries, where the cost of maternity benefits is shared by both the employer and the government. The increased cost of maternity benefits following the amended 2017 Act increases the potential for discrimination of female employees of child-bearing age by employers. To avail maternity benefits, woman employees must have worked in an establishment of the employer for a period of at least 80 days during the 12 months immediately preceding the date of her expected delivery. There is evidence that employers are potentially manipulating women's working conditions to ensure that they do not qualify for maternity entitlements. In the annual report of the National Commission for Women 2017, several complaints were reported from women across India whose maternity leave or other benefits had been denied by their employers. The impacted women were typically employed on contractual, temporary, daily wage, informal, or ad hoc basis in various government and private organizations.

Despite lower wages and fewer opportunities when compared to men, women are increasingly entering the workforce in India, Pakistan, and Bangladesh. Bangladesh historically has had low participation rates by women working outside of the household. In recent years, the number of jobs available to women within the textile industry has increased in both the domestic and export market. Workers employed in Bangladesh export-processing zones (EPZ) tend to receive pay and benefits that closely resembled those of the formal sector. These included paid vacation and maternity leave, overtime pay, medical care at work, and childcare facilities. Kabeer (2012) however reports that women take on paid work in addition to working in the home, thus adding to their overall work burden and consequently leading to burnout and stress.

In 2005, the Indian Parliament passed the National Rural Employment Guarantee Act (NREGA) legislation. The NREGA is a national law funded largely by the central government in India and implemented in all states in the country, which creates a "right to work" for all households in rural India. Under the NREGA, households in rural India have a legal right to get "at least" 100 days of unskilled manual labor in each financial year which, as per law, is to be provided by local government when work is demanded by any worker or group of workers registered under the NREGA. NREGA facilitates women's empowerment by providing opportunities to obtain paid employment. Three key provisions for women in the Act are: (1) a third of all employment is reserved for women; (2) there must be provision of childcare facilities at the workplace; and (3) both men and women must receive the statutory state government minimum wage. The employment works operated under the NREGA in India have had a significant impact on the lives of women workers. Khera and Nayak (2009) reported that over half NREGA workers used their wages to treat an illness within the family. The scheme has resulted in women accessing higher wages which has improved the health and lives of their children. The scheme has also been credited with allowing women to collect and keep their own wage and positively impact the lives of children. However, the implementation of the scheme differs across Indian states. Khera and Nayak (2009) also reported that in some states childcare services were unavailable and that the scheme only applies to the rural sector of the economy and provides employment for a minimum of 100 days a year.

Table 5.3 Retirement age and share of parliament seats for women versus men in South Asian countries

	Bangladesh		India		Pakistan	
	Women	Men	Women	Men	Women	Men
Statutory retirement age in 2015	60	60	55	55	55	60
Proportion of seats held by women in national parliaments in 2018	20.3%	79.7%	11.8%	88.2%	20.6%	79.4%

Source: This data has been retrieved from publically available data-sets by STATISTA

Two key indicators for the value and enabling power of women of South Asia, in relation to employment, are presented in Table 5.3. We can see that working women retire early at 55 and 60 years, respectively, in India and Bangladesh. Women in Pakistan are forced to retire 5 years before men, at 55 years. This means that women working in the formal sector have less provident fund and less health coverage years from employers. In all three countries, women are critically underrepresented in parliament (Bangladesh = 20.3%; India = 11.8%; and Pakistan = 20.6%). The fewer the women in parliament, the less likelihood that women can mobilize change for their own gender's employment conditions, such as: (i) formal sector work participation; (ii) protection for unskilled, home-based, and agricultural workers; (iii) labor laws and minimum wages; (iv) workplace safety and harassment laws; and (iii) employment benefits like leave with pay, health insurance, and specifically maternity benefits.

5.4 Access to Healthcare for South Asian Women: Informal Sector Workers and Non-workers

According to the National Family Health Survey of India carried out between 2015 and 2016, NFHS-4, the percentage of households with at least one family member covered by a health scheme or by health insurance has increased from 4.8% in 2005 to 28.7% in 2016. However, due to the critical problem of lack of access for majority population, a scheme called Ayushman Bharat Yojana was launched under the Ministry of Health and Family Welfare in India, which aims to provide health coverage to half a billion individuals by 2022 (Ayushman Bharat 2018). Key targets for the scheme include:

1. Shifting focus from "sick-care" to "wellness" by promoting prevention and well-being.
2. Increasing healthcare access and quality at reduced cost to patients. The scheme proposes free drugs and diagnostics as well as free emergency and essential healthcare services in public hospitals.
3. The policy targets to reduce preventable mortality of non-communicable diseases by advocating pre-screening.
4. Promotion of "Make in India" initiative using drugs and devices manufactured in India.

A plan to achieve universal health coverage (UHC) in Bangladesh by 2032 was announced by Prime Minister Sheikh Hasina in 2011. A study carried out by El-Saharty et al. (2015) identified several challenges facing Bangladesh in achieving UHC by 2032. There is a severe shortage of qualified health professionals within Bangladesh. This is due to low salaries in the public sector, migration of healthcare professionals overseas, and difficulties of staff retention in remote areas. A gender imbalance exists within the health profession. Low status of the nursing profession leads to a shortage of workers and increased pressure on staff working within the health sector. Within the country, an urban bias exists in relation to healthcare. Fewer than 20% of healthcare professionals provide services to more than 75 percent of the rural population. The doctor-to-population ratio is 10 times worse in rural areas (1:15,000) compared to urban areas (1:1,500). The authors conclude that the challenges facing UHC in Bangladesh can be addressed by: (i) accelerated hiring for current vacancies, (ii) increasing recruitment of nurses, and (iii) increasing the status of the healthcare professionals in Bangladesh through financial and non-financial incentives.

Similarly, there is no universal health coverage in Pakistan, with serious shortages in health resources and staffing. Cultural barriers prevent women from accessing services from male practitioners. A report by the BBC in 2017 highlighted that although 70% of all medical students in Pakistan are women, there is a shortage of practicing women doctors within the country (BBC 2017). Many women doctors in Pakistan are unable to continue their careers post-marriage due to cultural barriers and lack of support from their family. Two women doctors were motivated to launch Sehat Kahani, a Telehealth company utilizing technology to provide health services to women patients. The women doctors working with Sehat Kahani conduct online medical consultations to treat patients who visit the healthcare centers. This model has increased access to affordable, effective healthcare to low-income women and their families in rural areas, urban slums, and middle income communities of Pakistan. However, it is not accessible for women patients without technology and can never be a replacement for physical checkups, diagnosis, and interventions.

The ability of women to access healthcare was studied by Bloom et al. (2001) using a sample of 300 women from Varanasi, India. Their study showed that in South Asia women's autonomy is as important a factor in access to healthcare as education. Women who were allowed by husband and in-laws to maintain close connections to their natal kin had increased health access, as they had support from their parents and siblings for time, transport, and finances. It was also found that women with greater social and geographical mobility obtained higher levels of antenatal care. Thus, there is a complex cultural problem in South Asia that even when health resources and practitioners may become widely available, it is the cultural and social support that needs to be improved for health benefits to women. This implies that interventions for women's development and health improvements must include simultaneous social awareness and cultural reform agendas.

5.5 Microfinance and Health Access for Women Borrowers

Microcredit is the extension of very small loans, microloans, to impoverished borrowers who typically lack collateral, steady employment, or a verifiable credit history. It is designed to support entrepreneurship and alleviate poverty. Modern microcredit is generally considered to have originated with the Grameen Bank founded in Bangladesh in 1983. Microcredit organizations were initially created as alternatives to the "loan sharks" known to take advantage of clients through high interest rate on loans. Microcredit is part of microfinance, which provides a wider range of financial services, especially savings accounts, to the poor. Small-scale financial services improve the income ability of disadvantaged people, in particular, women. The main reason cited for a preference for lending to women are lower default rates on loans and higher likelihood that loan benefits the wider family. Microfinance institutions (MFIs) facilitate access to credit for women, allowing them greater independence, the ability to invest in their businesses, and increased earning and spending power. As a consequence, women are better able to provide for their families, with regard to food, education, and health. MFIs engage in group lending where loans are issued to a group of clients, referred to as a self-help group (SHGs) instead of to individual clients. Members of the SHG share the responsibility for loan repayment with the group collectively deciding how the loan is allocated to group members.

For many, microfinance is a way to promote economic development, employment, and growth through the support of micro-entrepreneurs and small businesses; for others, it is a way for the poor to manage their finances more effectively and take advantage of economic opportunities while managing the risks. Terminology used within the sector has evolved over time – from microcredit to microfinance and now "financial inclusion." There are substantial claims in the literature that MFIs enable women to invest in small businesses and take care of their families and that microfinance is an effective instrument for poverty alleviation and women's empowerment (Kodamarty 2016). Loomba analyzed the performance of SHGs in Uttar Pradesh, India, and reported a significant improvement in participants' incomes after joining SHGs. Group members reported increased economic and social empowerment, a greater role in decision-making within the family.

The impact of women's autonomy and gender relations after participation in microcredit programs in Bangladesh is considered by Pitt et al. (2003). The authors analyzed a dataset collected in a qualitative study of 1798 households from 87 villages carried out in rural Bangladesh in 1999 where 905 of the 1798 households participate in a credit program. Participation by women within microcredit programs was found to help increase women's empowerment, leading to women having a greater say in decisions related to the household. In contrast, the effect of men's participation in group-based credit was found to have a neutral to negative impact, reducing their wives' ability to travel, access financial resources, and contribute in decision-making.

The challenge with the use of microfinance lies in the creation of credit instruments that meet the credit requirements of low-income borrowers without resulting in too high transaction costs for the MFIs. Agarwal (2016) notes that group lending which utilizes self-help groups (SHGs), while effective in leveraging the social collateral that low-income borrowers have access to, comes at the risk of increased stress and pressure which can disempower women borrowers.

Khan and Noreen (2012) analyzed data from 600 female clients from 2 MFIs operating in the Southern Punjab district of Pakistan over the period 2002–2007 to identify factors significant to determining female empowerment. Marital status, age, and number of children of the microfinance client were more significant factors in explaining empowerment as compared with access to and control over microfinance loans. In the perspective of woman empowerment, the authors recommended microfinance institutions perform checks to determine whether the loans were being utilized by the woman borrowers themselves (or their family members) and offer additional management and vocational training to women borrowers as a means of supporting their empowerment.

The literature from Bangladesh suggests that microfinance initiatives from NGOs do not have any programs for the extreme poor (Khatun et al. 2013). Many women borrowers from the extreme poor group who had dropped out from MFIs reported being discouraged from taking out a microfinance loan for a variety of reasons, including: (i) weekly repayments with high interest rates are a major deterrent that discouraged borrowers, (ii) the loan amounts on offer were very small, and borrowers were unable to set up businesses using the amount of credit on offer, (iii) several women borrowers reported obtaining credit only for their husbands where the funds were spent by them on discretionary spending; (iv) several women borrowers interviewed reported experiencing mental stress as a result of struggling to repay the loans; and (v) too many long meetings regarding bureaucratic process.

People who are extremely poor do not have many safety nets to fall back on. The likelihood of high downside risk associated with defaulting on loans at high interest rates acts as a deterrent on women borrowers. Women borrowers are deterred by the increased uncertainty and downside risk. Not taking on the loan was preferred because it avoids the risk of mental stress that is experienced by the bank borrower on loan default. Non-members of MFIs were deterred by high interest rates and the difficulty that they expected in trying to repay the loan. Some of the people surveyed expressed no desire of a loan. Some non-members reported that they were prevented from doing so by their husbands. From the group of extreme poor, NGOs reported that in a high percentage of cases loans were misused. Instead, loans often end up being misused by borrowers, for family consumption, social function, or ending up being lent to others. No follow-up services were provided by NGO-MFIs to members in the activities undertaken with the loans.

In 2011, 59% of microfinance loans in Pakistan were made to women, a lower participation rate compared to other South Asian countries. A large percentage of loans made to women appeared to be passed onto male members of the household instead of being used directly by the female borrowers. The presence of credit information bureaus results in men who previously defaulted on loans gaining access to credit through women (Safavian and Haq 2013). A study by Safavian and Haq (2013) identified several reasons for low MFI loan uptake by female entrepreneurs in Pakistan: (1) usual approach of microfinance loans occurs via group lending instead of allowing individual loans to be made. The majority of loan participants would prefer individual loans. (2) Inadequate loan size and high transaction costs (form filling and documentation requirements, meeting attendance, travel costs) raised the loan cost beyond the repayment of interest rate. (3) Requirement for unrelated males to act as loan guarantors and approval is required by male household heads. Lending to young unmarried women without a guarantor was regarded as highly risky by MFIs.

Several microfinance institutions (MFIs) in South Asia offer health insurance schemes in conjunction with their loans. By using the existing rural networks of the MFI, the programs have lower transaction costs. Healthcare and microfinance are interrelated with borrowers often using microfinance loans or savings for health expenditures. Roth et al. (2005) argue in favor of commercialization of microinsurance, noting that a variety of products and services including insurance products are required by the poor to manage effectively. Without support from the MFIs, many of the poor in South Asia end up borrowing from moneylenders to meet expenses and get trapped in a debt cycle. A large portion of the outstanding debts of poor women are used for healthcare. Roth et al. (2005) compared the various microinsurance products available to the poor, such as those for life insurance, property, endowment, agriculture, and health insurance available from three different microfinance institutions, highlighting their advantages and disadvantages to the policy holders. They note a number of challenges to commercializing microinsurance such as reducing transactions costs; managing adverse selection, moral hazard, fraud, and overusage; creating an enabling regulatory environment; developing sustainable health products; and overcoming natural resistance to purchasing insurance and educational barriers.

Rai and Ravi (2011) assessed the claims behavior of borrowers and their spouses, with the goal of understanding how microfinance, gender, and health insurance interact. They used a data set consisting of 280,000 microfinance borrowers in India who were required to purchase health insurance once they obtained a loan. Their main finding was that borrowers make considerably more use of health insurance (in terms of filing their claims) than their partners do. Moreover, women who are borrowers make significantly more use of health insurance than non-borrowing women who have obtained the insurance through their spouses, supporting the view that microfinance empowers women. Ill health impacts the ability of MFI clients to repay their loans and flourish in their microenterprise endeavors. The cost of medical treatment can result in MFI clients using microfinance loans and assets to pay for medical treatment. The barriers of healthcare costs, accessibility of healthcare services, cultural practices, and lack of trust in healthcare professionals can reduce usage of healthcare services by the poor. Leatherman et al. (2011) identified several areas in which MFI can assist in improving their client's health. The first area is in the provision of health, sanitation, and nutrition education to MFI clients. This training is relatively straightforward to deliver and can result in behavior change which reduces the likelihood of illness.

A second approach is for MFIs to partner with local healthcare providers in rural areas. MFIs often will not have medical professions among their staff, so it is often more cost-effective for them to partner with healthcare providers in the community. A third area of assistance that MFIs can facilitate is in increasing access to health products by trained village entrepreneurs who can sell health products and medicines and provide education to the local community. The activities of these entrepreneurs should be supervised and their efficacy measured to ensure sound practices. Healthcare financing and microinsurance are another means by which MFIs can assist their clients. The MFI can leverage their existing networks to provide a cost-effective insurance solutions. Regulation is required to ensure that the products offered are properly priced and regulated. As the insurance sector is different to the banking sector, MFIs should employ actuaries to help ensure that insurance products are correctly priced. There is a need for regulation of the insurance products offered by MFIs.

Adding healthcare products can help MFIs improve client loyalty and competitive advantage. NRSP Microfinance Bank is a microfinance bank in Pakistan offering complimentary health insurance product to all of its microcredit clients and their spouse. The offer of health insurance covers hospitalization, accidental death, and disability of microcredit to clients and their spouses. The health insurance premium is factored into the loan interest rate charged to bank borrower (microcredit loan's interest rates were 30% in September 2019). There is evidence in the literature of dissatisfaction with the health insurance products that are combined with microfinance lending (Safavian and Haq 2013). Borrowers report that they would not buy the health insurance product if it was not compulsory with the loan. In some cases, the concept of insurance was not well understood by policyholders, and there was mistrust of continued payment of an insurance premium without any claims being made. Often health insurance schemes require policyholders to pay at the time of treatment and subsequently request a claim from the policy providers. This process can deter policyholders from obtaining treatment if they do not have money to pay; further the responsibility lies with the policyholder to follow up and make payment for treatment. Life insurance produces were viewed as a saving scheme and were more favorably received.

5.6 Breaking the Cycle of Generational Poverty

In this part of the chapter, we discuss three examples of programs run in Bangladesh, India, and Pakistan with the goal of reaching and improving the lives of the Ultra Poor.

5.6.1 Bangladesh: BRAC – CFPR-TUP Program

Challenging the Frontiers of Poverty Reduction: Targeting the Ultra Poor (CFPR-TUP) is a project started in 2002 by BRAC, a Bangladesh-based development organization. The ultra poor constitutes the poorest, that is, 17.6% of the population of Bangladesh (HIES 2010). The CFPR-TUP program is focused on families who are too poor to access the benefits from development interventions such as microfinance and assists them to access mainstream development services. The services provided by CFPR-TUP program to its clients include asset and cash transfers, healthcare, social integration, livelihood development training, and hands-on coaching for 24 months to build confidence and graduate them out of ultra-poverty. A study carried out by Das and Misha (2010) found that more than 95% of participants in the CFPR program left the category of ultra-poverty over the 2-year program, and they had successfully remained out of poverty 4 years on. Bandiera and colleagues (2013) performed a control trial in 2013 and found increases in the value of livestock, employment, and earnings of CFPR program participants well after the formal program had ended.

Despite the gains of the CFPR-TUP, we must consider three important findings. One, that because the program has been limited to only three poor districts (Rangpur, Kurigram, and NNilphamari), there are limited benefits for poor women across the country. A successful pilot effort such as CFPR-TUP must be replicated across the country for wider and sustainable impact. Second, there is evidence that participants of the program suffered from increased health expenses and had to forgo more working days due to illness. This implies that perhaps additional workload and pressure to generate income has a detrimental effect on health quality of life and there is need of simultaneous support in income generation activities and healthcare in impoverished populations. Last, in the long term, primary enrollment for boys in participant families was noted. This implies that there are still critical cultural barriers to girls' education even when household income increases.

5.6.2 Pakistan: Benazir Income Support Program (BISP)

The Benazir Income Support Program (BISP) is a social assistance program in Pakistan serving over five million people. The program was launched in 2008 by the Government of Pakistan with the objective to provide a social protection floor to the poorest section of society by providing them unconditional cash transfers (UCT). As of July 2015, the monthly value of the payment per family was PKR 1566/USD 10.1.[1] In order to increase women's empowerment within the family, BISP payments are made to the female head of beneficiary households. Cash transfer is made quarterly, with the vast majority of beneficiaries now receiving cash through the

[1] Currency conversion: https://www.xe.com/currencyconverter/

BISP Debit Card. The program has also created BISP Beneficiary Committees (BBC) that provide a forum for beneficiaries. The cash transfer targets the poorest 25% of the population, and eligible program participants are identified using a scorecard with a specific eligibility threshold for the BISP UCT.

Cheema and Hunt et al. (2016) found that the BISP UCT has influenced a change in the way women are viewed in the household and in the community. Beneficiary women interviewed reported that they were given an elevated status within the household as a direct result of the BISP UCT program. The program also increased the mobility and independence of women, with female participants allowed to travel unaccompanied within their communities. However, there have been serious criticisms against the BISP including: (i) release of funds to the non-poor, (ii) inability of UCT to match hyperinflation in the country, (iii) the program was federally administered and was unable to reach most of the disadvantaged populations across the provinces, and (iv) administrative faults such as inability to monitor double counting and control operational costs (Ahmad 2018). The new government has now replaced the program with another poverty alleviation scheme in 2019, the impact of which cannot be assessed.

5.6.3 India: Parinaam Foundation

Parinaam Foundation is a not-for-profit organization founded in 2008 to cater to the educational and healthcare needs of the urban poor in India. The different programs piloted by the foundation over the years include (i) health camps, (ii) financial literacy programs, (iii) ultra poor program, and (iv) academic adoption program. Parinaam trialed various health schemes including outpatient services, medicine, and health camps followed by a move to more specialized treatment for ENT and Dental. Approximately 500–600 customers attended each health camp. The findings were that it was difficult for patients to follow up due to lack of time and travel for treatment. In the absence of extreme pain, people tended to delay or avoid treatment. Currently, patients tend to borrow money from family to pay for medical treatment. As such, health camps were found to be relatively inefficient in improving healthcare among the population and were stopped. The slow uptake of health insurance in India is due to preference to use state and government benefits.

The Diksha financial literacy program provides knowledge and tools to low-income families in India in order to save safely, reduce financial risk, and make informed financial decisions. Financial literacy is provided through a 5-week classroom training program. Program participants are also assisted to open savings bank accounts, and those that require credit facilities are linked to Ujjivan Bank, gaining access to financial products such as cashless facilities and individual loans. Diksha has assisted over 370,000 economically underprivileged women since its inception. The program is run across 20 states and union territories in India and is taught in 12 different languages.

In 2009, Parinaam piloted the Urban Ultra Poor program in Bengaluru, which majorly consists of migrant populations. A total of 5000 families have taken part in the program since 2009. Parinaam involvement with families is initially for a 1-year period. During this period, there is an initial set of weekly meetings with families taking part in the program. Financial services provided to participants include how to use ATM machines, how to deposit and withdraw money, and how to manage a bank account. Though the intention was to improve business activities, the feedback received from program participants is that they are reluctant to setting up businesses and being self-employed and instead prefer to take support in finding higher paid employment. Healthcare provided to participants includes vaccines, twice yearly deworming, and the cost of medical interventions. Families are connected with pharmacies who provide a 20% discount on medicines. Parinaam conducts tuition centers run by field community works which engage children from the age of 4 to 14 years and introduces them to a formal hour of disciplined study time 6 days a week. The children are enrolled into the closest government schools or Anganwadi schools to resume education. Through the years, the committed students are tracked and moved into Parinaam's Academic Adoption Program.

Parinaam's Academic Adoption Program (AAP) provides access to high quality education to children from low-income families through a sponsorship scheme. As of 2019, the program has sponsored the education of 600 children. As part of the program, health insurance is provided for up to seven siblings of the student and their mother. The cover includes cover for hospital visits up to 1 lakh rupees as well as five medical treatments costing up to 1500 rupees per year. The premium charged for health insurance is 2120 rupees per family with 1000 rupees of the premium paid for by the family and the remainder subsidized by the Parinaam Foundation. The main challenge reported by health insurance policyholders is that participants do not understand the hospital claim process. Overall, the major issue facing Parinaam Foundation is how to widen services and reach all the poor in India. There are limitations in reachability and impact as the Foundation is dependent on volunteers and donations and cannot compare with the benefits, or access and impact, of a government administered program.

Case Study from Pakistan: Is Poverty Emergence Possible without Support for Health and Nutrition?

The aim was to understand the health quality of life of borrowers after loan-taking for small business development. This is a summary of an interview with a poor woman borrower from Hyderabad Sindh. Najma (name has been changed to preserve anonymity) has been issued a loan amount of PKR 100,000/USD 644.7 for 1 year and is paying PKR 10,000/USD 64.5 back per month at an interest rate of 10% from a local microfinance bank, regulated by the State Bank of Pakistan. She is a 24-year-old married housewife with three

(continued)

daughters. Najma is also responsible for providing care to one dependent aging family member unable to physically do all their tasks themselves.

Najma and her family live in considerable poverty, earning PKR 40,000/ USD 257.9 per month. The loan is being used by her husband to pay rent for a shop where he sells cloth purchased from a bigger local cloth vendor. Najma and her husband are first time borrowers in the 8th month of a 12-month loan schedule. Her husband pays the loan installment, and their monthly income is dependent on the sales made by her husband. The day her husband is not well and the shop is not opened is not a fortunate day for the family, as it usually means they only eat one meal that day.

On being asked which problems she and her family have faced since taking loans, Najma replied that they faced difficulty in repaying loans and that the duration of having to repay installments on a monthly basis was too short. She also described that household expenses are difficult to manage, with money not being enough for purchases related to food and medicine for household members, specifically children and aging parents. The two food items that Najma stated she could not afford to buy in the last 6 months were meat and fruit. On being asked which health problems she faced herself, Najma listed weight loss and lack of appetite. On being further questioned if she had sought medical consultancy and been advised any tests for these symptoms, Najma replied no. However, she hesitantly shared that she was taking a pregnancy multivitamin as she was expecting her fourth child and hoping for a son this time.

Najma's family was not receiving any health insurance from the microfinance provider or the government. Neither did the family have money for private uptake of a health insurance scheme. On being asked which health problems and expenses the family members faced in the last 6 months, the woman borrower stated infections and fever for the children and hypertension and aches and pains for the adults and elderly. The local government health center was available to access for health needs. However, the woman claimed that the center was not in a proper condition and there were no free medicines available for poor people. It was also mentioned that medical practitioners did not give complete information or discuss options for treatment. As a consequence, the woman stated that she mostly preferred to seek healthcare assistance from elders in the family or the local healer.

Though the woman's husband owned the house they lived in, seven family members shared two rooms in the house. There was no water connection and garbage disposal system accessible to them. As a result, Najma was responsible for collecting water from a local pump and carrying the garbage a distance from the house. Overall, the borrower was of the opinion that the loan had not helped her family emerge from poverty and that the stress of loan repayment added to their burden and troubles. The limitation of this narration

(continued)

is that the respondent is illiterate and is not utilizing the loan herself. Her answers are perception based, and she may not be reporting the exact amount of monthly household income and monthly loan repayment schedule. Much of the information that Najma is sharing is perception based and cannot be verified entirely, as is true with qualitative data. However, we learn important lessons from this case study. Small loans without health insurance schemes cannot guarantee emergence from poverty and improvement in quality of lives or health and well-being in poor women borrowers living in disadvantaged circumstances. Also, many women borrowers do not use loans for autonomous income-generating opportunities. Ethics approval for this study was taken from the Institutional Review Board, Forman Christian College University.

5.7 Conclusion

The iceberg of disease in women of South Asia will only be disclosed when health coverage is available and health access is optimal. The crippling dilemma of the feminization of poverty, perpetuated by regressive cultural forces and structural failure, have so far prevented women from accessing limited private healthcare services. Small-scale efforts have been made to help women emerge from poverty and access credit but they have not been as effective in empowering women holistically across the large expanse of South Asia for adequate poverty alleviation and health support. We strongly believe that there is need for replication of successful small poverty alleviation programs at state-level across South Asia. Similarly, though private foundations and microfinance providers are supporting some women for health relief, there is need to secure universal health insurance for women through the state to ensure access for all.

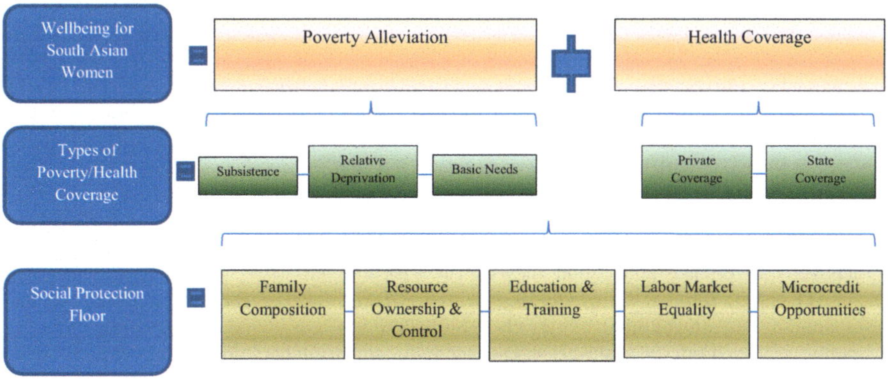

Fig. 5.1 Model describing a pathway for poverty alleviation and health coverage for women of South Asia

In Fig. 5.1, we summarize what we have learnt in this chapter and present a basic pathway for poverty alleviation and health coverage for the women of South Asia. We recommend more organized and systematic efforts to develop a dependable and sustainable social protection floor for women with features of: (i) support for basic needs for disadvantaged women groups, like single women households, the sick, and the disabled, including housing, sanitation, water, and food security; (ii) reform of cultural practices for inheritance and ownership of women; (iii) improvement in educational enrollment for girls and literacy and skill development for adult women; (iv) pulling women into the workforce and providing working women with formal sector employment benefits, including basic income, employment contracts and pension benefits, safety at workplace, leave with pay, and health and maternity benefits; and (v) providing small business opportunities through microcredit with consideration of nonfinancial social development features.

References

Agarwal, B. (2016). *Role of micro finance in empowering Indian women*. Available at http://www.icehm.org/upload/3749ED1116007.pdf

Ahmad, S. (2018). Can BISP be used for poverty reduction? *Journal of History Culture and Art Research, 7*(3), 713–723. https://doi.org/10.7596/taksad.v7i3.1643.

Ayushman Bharat. (2018). Source: https://pib.gov.in/PressReleaseIframePage.aspx?PRID=1518544

Bandiera, B., et al. (2013). *Can basic entrepreneurship transform the economic lives of the poor?*. (IZA discussion paper no. 7386). Source: SSRN: https://ssrn.com/abstract=2266813

BBC. (2017). *How to stop female doctors from dropping out in Pakistan*. BBC World Hacks. Source: https://www.bbc.co.uk/news/av/magazine-41003627/how-to-stop-female-doctors-from-dropping-out-in-pakistan

Bloom, Wypij, & Gupta. (2001). Dimensions of women's autonomy and the influence on maternal health care utilization in a North Indian city. *Demography, 38*, 67–78.

Cheema, Hunt, et al. (2016). *Benazir income support programme*. Oxford Policy Management. Source: https://www.opml.co.uk/files/Publications/7328-evaluating-pakistans-flagship-social-protection-programme-bisp/bisp-final-impact-evaluation-report.pdf?noredirect=1.

Cossman & Kapur. (1993). Women and poverty in India: Law and social change. *Canadian Journal of Women and the Law, 6*, 278.

Das, & Mehta. (2012). *Poverty and social exclusion in India: Women*. Washington, DC. World Bank. Source: https://openknowledge.worldbank.org/handle/10986/26338. License: CC BY 3.0 IGO.

Das, N., & Misha, F. (2010). *Addressing extreme poverty in a sustainable manner: Evidence from CFPR programme* (Working papers). esocialsciences.com.

Davis, P. (2011). *Escaping poverty: patterns and causes of poverty exits in rural Bangladesh*. Chronic Poverty Research Center May 2011, Working paper 194. Source: http://www.chronicpoverty.org/uploads/publication_files/WP194%20Davis.pdf

Dharam G. (1999). *Building knowledge organizations: Achieving excellence*. Unpublished excerpt. Source: https://web.archive.org/web/20140319063854/http://www.ilo.org/wcmsp5/groups/public/%2D%2D-dgreports/%2D%2D-dcomm/documents/genericdocument/wcms_193047.pdf

El-Saharty, Powers, et al. (2015). *The path to universal health coverage in Bangladesh: Bridging the gap of human resources for health* (World Bank study). Washington, DC: World Bank.

HIES. (2010). *Report of the household income and expenditure survey 2010*. Bangladesh Bureau of Statistics.

Hindu Succession (Amendment) Act. (2005). Source: https://www.hrln.org/admin/issue/subpdf/HSA_Amendment_2005.pdf

Holmes, Fouzia, et al. (2010). *Gendered risks, poverty and vulnerability in Bangladesh. Case study of the Challenging the Frontiers of Poverty Reduction programme (CFPR), Specially Targeted Ultra Poor II (STUP II)*. London: Overseas Development Institute.

ILO. (2010). *Women in labor markets: Measuring progress and identifying challenges*. Source: http://www.ilo.org/wcmsp5/groups/public/%2D%2D-ed_emp/%2D%2D-emp_elm/%2D%2D-trends/documents/publication/wcms_123835.pdf

ILO. (2011). Social security for social justice and a fair globalization: Recurrent discussion on social protection (social security) under the ILO Declaration ON Social Justice for a Fair Globalization Report VI, International Labour Conference, 100thSession, Geneva, 2011.

ILO. (2018). *World employment social outlook trends 2018*. International Labour Office. Source: http://www.ilo.org/wcmsp5/groups/public/%2D%2D-dgreports/%2D%2D-dcomm/%2D%2D-publ/documents/publication/wcms_615594.pdf

Kabeer, N. (2012). Between affiliation and autonomy: navigating pathways of women's empowerment and gender justice in Bangladesh. *Development and Change, 42*(2), 499–528.

Khan, & Noreen. (2012). Microfinance and women empowerment: A case study of district Bahawalpur (Pakistan). *African Journal of Business Management, 6*(12), 4514–4521.

Khatun, et al. (2013). Why some poor women in Bangladesh do not opt for micro-credit? *Journal of the Bangladesh Agricultural University, 11*(2), 285–292.

Khera, & Nayak. (2009). *Women workers and perceptions of the NREGA*. Source: https://core.ac.uk/download/pdf/2790414.pdf

Ki-Moon, B. (2010). *Global strategy for women's and children's health*. New York: United Nations.

Kodamarty. (2016). Microfinance and women empowerment: Self perception of beneficiaries – A study with reference to Gandhinagar District of Gujarat. *Indian Journal of Applied Research, 6*(2).

Leatherman, et al. (2011). *Integrating microfinance and health benefits, challenges and reflections for moving forward*. Source: https://www.freedomfromhunger.org/integrating-microfinance-and-health-benefits-challenges-and-reflections-moving-forward

Lipton, M. (1986). *Seasonality and Ultrapoverty* (IDS Bulletin 17.3). Institute of Development Studies. Source: http://www.ids.ac.uk/files/dmfile/Lipton17.3final.pdf

MBA (1961). The Maternity Benefit Act, India 1961. https://www.ilo.org/dyn/travail/docs/678/maternitybenefitsact1961.pdf

MBAA (2017). Maternity Benefit (Amendment) Act 2017. https://www.ilo.org/dyn/natlex/natlex4.detail?p_lang=en&p_isn=106425&p_count=1&p_classification=16

National Commission for Women. (2017). *Annual report 2017–2018*. Source: http://ncw.nic.in/sites/default/files/ANNUALREPORT2017_18.pdf

National Statistical Commission. (2012). *Government of India*. Report of the Committee on Unorganised Sector Statistics.

NFHS-4. The National Family Health Survey. (2015a–2016). *(NFHS-4), Indian Ministry of Health and Family Welfare. Key indicators*. Source: http://rchiips.org/nfhs/pdf/NFHS4/India.pdf

NFHS-4. The National Family Health Survey. (2015b–2016). *Ministry of Health and Family Welfare*. Source: http://rchiips.org/nfhs/pdf/NFHS4/India.pdf

Panda, & Agarwal. (2005). Marital violence, human development and women's property status in India. *World Development, 33*(5), 823–850.

Pitt, M., et al. (2003). *Does micro-credit empower women? Evidence from Bangladesh*. Washington, DC: The World Bank Development Research Group Rural Development.

Rai, & Ravi. (2011). Do spouses make claims? Female empowerment and microfinance. *World Development, 39*(6), 913–921.

Roth, Raman, & Namerta. (2005). *Microinsurance and microfinance institutions – Evidence from India*. CGAP Working Group on Micro insurance, Good and Bad Practices, Case Study No.15, September.

Safavian, M., & Haq, A. (2013). *Are Pakistan's women entrepreneurs being served by the microfinance sector? Directions in development*. Washington, DC: World Bank.

Selvaratnam, S. (1988). Population and status of women. *Asia-Pacific Population Journal, 3*(2), 3–28.

Siddiqui, R., & Hamid, S. (2009). *Correlates of poverty: Gender dimensions*. Study prepared for IDRC, Canada in collaboration with ISST, India.

SPF Advisory Group. (2011). *Social protection floor for a fair and inclusive globalization (Bachelet report)*. Geneva: International Labour Office.

Srivastava, R. S. (2013). *A social protection floor for India*. New Delhi: International Labour Office, ILO DWT for South Asia and ILO Country Office for India.

Townsend, P. (2006, December). What is poverty? An historical perspective. In *Poverty in focus* (pp. 5–6). Brasilia: United Nations Development Programme, International Poverty Centre.

Umme, & Malik. (2012). *Why highly educated women face potential poverty: A case study in Dhaka, Bangladesh*. Bangladesh Development Research Working Paper Series (BDRWPS).

United Nations. (2000). *Report of the Ad Hoc Committee of the Whole of the twenty-third special session of the General Assembly* (A/S-23/10/Rev.1). New York: United Nations.

WEF. (2018). *The global gender gap report 2018*. World Economic Forum. Source: http://www3.weforum.org/docs/WEF_GGGR_2018.pdf.

WHO. (2005). *Medical costs push millions of people into poverty across the globe*, 5 December 2005. Source: http://www.who.int/mediacentre/news/releases/2005/pr65/en/

Chapter 6
Refugee, Displaced, and Climate-Affected Women of South Asia and Their Health Challenges

Sara Rizvi Jafree and Bajiyanta Mukhopadhyay

6.1 Introduction

South Asia is suffering from sustained political mismanagement, ethnic conflict, natural disasters, and environmental degradation. Nearly 50 million refugees have crossed borders in South Asia since the colonial rule ended. By the end of 2018, more than 15% of the world's total disasters and more than 5% of the total world conflict were reported in South Asia (IDMC 2018). This has led to a familiar and widespread culture of displacement and marginalization in the region, which civilians and governing bodies have become immune to. Environmental disasters and regional conflict have a definite gender bias with women suffering much more compared to the men. As shown in Table 6.1, UNHCR reports the South Asian figures for women refugees, IDPs, and forced migrants due to conflict or climate change, at an estimated 10.3 million, with more women being reported than men (UNHCR 2018). However, there is extreme uncertainty of determining updated figures due to the complexity of constant fluidity and change in population flow caused by geopolitical stress (Marbach 2018).

Since the 1960s, the number of displaced women has increased compared to men (United Nations Development Programme 2009). This feminization of displacement has brought to attention that women compared to men during and after migration are not equal, and women face considerable challenges in health experiences due to greater emotional and physical burdens and also due to greater vulnerabilities from violence and sexual abuse. As there is no health data set available especially

S. R. Jafree
Department of Sociology, Forman Christian College University, Lahore, Pakistan

B. Mukhopadhyay (✉)
Cree Board of Health and Social Services, Waskaganish, Canada

Department of Family Medicine, McGill University, Montreal, Canada

S. R. Jafree (ed.), *The Sociology of South Asian Women's Health*,
https://doi.org/10.1007/978-3-030-50204-1_6

Table 6.1 Women refugees, IDPs, and migrants, 2018, UNHCR[a]

	Total	Women[c]	Percentage of women from total
Refugees and IDPs (UNHCR 2018)[b]			
Afghanistan	2,537,063	1,340,490	53%
Bangladesh	943,375	473,540	50%
India	208,301	18,562	9%
Nepal	21,605	10,941	51%
Myanmar[d]	862,896	430,000	50%
Pakistan	1,580,046	736,669	47%
Sri Lanka	36,269	1308	4%
Total refugees and IDPs	**6,189,555**	**3,011,510**	**49%**
Migrants[e]			
Afghanistan	133,612	25,128	19%
Bangladesh	1,500,921	405,520	27%
Bhutan	52,296	4398	8%
India	5,188,550	3,578,808	69%
Maldives	67,026	3912	6%
Nepal	502,670	304,008	60%
Pakistan	3,398,154	2,943,824	87%
Sri Lanka	40,018	18,138	45%
Total migrants	**10,883,247**	**7,283,736**	**67%**
Total displaced populations	**17,072,802**	**10,295,246**	**60%**

[a]These figures include asylum-seekers, returnee refugees and IDPs, and stateless persons
[b]This data has been retrieved from publically available data-sets by UNHCR, source: https://www.unhcr.org/figures-at-a-glance.html
[c]This data has been retrieved from publically available data-sets by UNHCR, source: http://popstats.unhcr.org/en/demographics
[d]The nation-level figure for women was not available and thus an estimate by authors has been used based on population weightage
[e]This data has been retrieved from publically available data-sets by UN, source: https://www.un.org/en/development/desa/population/migration/data/estimates2/estimates17.asp

for women refugees and migrants, researchers have been depending on women's data sources for estimations, including household surveys, demographic health surveys, the living standards measurement surveys, and records of health institutions. Different variables from data sets have been used to determine health statistics for displaced women, such as "women's length of stay," "women's date of entry in country or region," and "women's citizenship status." However, there are major problems with this, such as (i) missing data from South Asian regions due to lack of access, conflict, and political barriers, (ii) missing variables in the data set as the surveys are not aimed to collect data on health issues of women displaced populations, and (iii) exclusion of temporary housing or shelters from the sample. Understandably, due to the lack of central and longitudinal data collection for women's health impacts caused by displacement, there is critical underestimation of needs and consequent policy making.

Climate change is the biggest threat to sustained gender inequality in health and is expected to worsen the divide between the Global North and Global South (Preet et al. 2010). Projections by the Intergovernmental Panel on Climate Change indicates that South Asian countries will face greater global warming and climate change compared to other countries of the world. Monsoon rain and the frequency of intense precipitation are predicted to increase, leading to flooding and droughts, which have multiple health consequences (Ahmed and Suphachalasai 2014). Not only are injuries and death caused by the effects of global warming, but flooding and droughts are a cause for damage and destruction of hospitals, clinics, and health centers. Furthermore, road blockages can prevent access to distant health services and trained practitioners. The direct impact of disease and abuse after climate change on women is substantial, but overall it also worsens their physical and emotional workload. In a region like South Asia, where the economies have been unable to prioritize women's economic participation and formal sector employment, the setbacks caused by climate change, till present day and as expected in the future, will further aggravate the case of gender-based equalities. The negligible policies that are being planned to mitigate the health consequences from climate change and conflict are also gender-blind, especially in the patriarchal and feudal regions of South Asia.

Women's demographic changes and realities related to displacement and climate change are also a concern. From the gendered demographic data that is available, in Table 6.2, it can be seen that majority of women migrants are above the age of 40 years (UN Population Division 2017). Thus, we not only have a problem of the feminization of displacement and migration, but we need to consider that due to the aging demographic composition of displaced women populations in South Asia, there would be greater demand for geriatric health attention. Though mortality rates and policy to reduce mortality is more discussed, there may also be a hidden issue

Table 6.2 Women international migration in South Asia by age, 2017, UNHCR

	Years					
Country	0–9	10–19	20–39	40–59	60+	Total
Afghanistan	3187	4579	11,679	4368	1315	25,128
Bangladesh	40,694	115,566	217,017	26,078	6165	405,520
Bhutan	487	427	2049	1077	358	4398
India	45,981	227,061	1,132,319	934,866	1,238,581	3,578,808
Maldives	530	457	1757	893	275	3912
Nepal	13,341	39,865	154,607	69,634	26,561	304,008
Pakistan	47,615	235,145	1,172,646	968,160	520,258	2,943,824
Sri Lanka	979	653	3663	7542	5301	18,138
South Asia	**152,814**	**623,753**	**2,695,737**	**2,012,618**	**1,798,814**	**7,283,736**
Percentage breakdown of age brackets	*2.1%*	*8.6%*	*37.0%*	*27.6%*	*24.7%*	*100%*

Source: This data has been retrieved from publically available data-sets by UN, source: https://www.un.org/en/development/desa/population/migration/data/estimates2/estimates17.asp

of reproductive burdens on South Asian displaced women and multiple births. Though there are no certain statistics, there is great cultural pressure on women for the birth of multiple male children fueled by regional uncertainty and environmental insecurity in displaced families. During times of poverty and hardships, many South Asian families are known to try for more children to gain more helping hands, placing immense reproductive pressure on women.

South Asian countries have the complexity of being both source and destination states for refugees and migrants (WHO South-East Asia Region 2018). The vulnerability of migration and displacement is a cause of serious physical and mental health consequences, which are more critical for women than men. Afghanistan faces a major displacement crisis due to years of war and internal conflict instigated by the terrorist group Taliban. Women especially are suffering health consequences due to extreme victimization and violence caused by Talibanization and war. Many women have become refugees and forced migrants in neighboring countries in order to escape from social deprivation, lack of health rights, extreme violence, and sexual slavery (Roshan 2004). The tripartite agreements by neighboring governments of Pakistan and Iran are attempting to assist Afghan refugees back to their own country; however, many women are reluctant to return due to fear of safety for themselves and their daughters. Though conditions as non-citizens living in refugee camps of Pakistan and Iran are not conducive to holistic well-being, Afghan refugee women still prefer to live as refugees rather than return home.

The country plagued by the highest rates of natural disasters in the world is Bangladesh, with many of the South Asian displaced populations belonging to this country. The women of the country have suffered more than the men for decades as greater burdens of livelihood and land recovery after disasters have been piled on their shoulders, without providing them relief from domestic and child responsibilities. For this reason, Bangladeshi women are also known to have unfavorable maternal health status and grave undernutrition (Hasan et al. 2017). Bangladesh with its own IDP problems, caused by natural disasters, is also the primary host for a large number of Rohingya refugees from Myanmar. India has one of the highest internal migration rates in the world due to ethnic conflict. Most migrants are without rights and health privileges as they are not considered citizens or ethnic natives of the destination areas. Without homes, jobs, and social acceptance, there are multiple health challenges facing the population, especially the women. India is also one of the least safe countries in the world for women to be living in, with displaced women being at higher risk of physical and sexual exploitation (Chhabra 2018). There is also the case of displaced Kashmiri women, who continue to bear the burden of longstanding repression by the government of India that limits the civil, political, social, and economic rights, coupled with the brute force of intense militarization. The tight control over data emerging from Kashmir makes it difficult to quantify the health impacts of Indian policy in Kashmir on displaced women.

Myanmar, like Bangladesh, has one of the highest rates of natural disasters, leading to internal displacement and forced migration since many decades. In addition, since 2017 there has been a humanitarian crisis with ethnic cleansing and extreme violence against the Rohingya Muslims in the Rakhine state. A mass exodus of

Rohingya refugees have been fleeing to Bangladesh and living in slum-like shelters in deplorable conditions. Rohingya women have been greater victims in terms of not just loss of homes but loss of dignity and well-being caused by high rates of violence and sexual assault (Hasan-ul-Bari and Ahmed 2018). Armed conflict between the Myanmar army and rebel groups in the Kachin, Chin, and Shan states has also contributed to IDPs in the country. Nepal, along with India, has been host to refugees from Tibet after the forced takeover by China. Oppression against the Tibetan Buddhist community has been recorded, but there has also been grave violence against the women, including women nuns (Härkönen 2016). Many IDPs also remain unsettled in Nepal due to the Maoist insurgency, communal violence in the Terai region, and the 2015 earthquakes. Displaced women in Nepal have been suffering from deprivation in basic health needs, discrimination, and sexual exploitation (Khatiwada and Bakhundol 2010).

Pakistan primarily faces great internal migration due to a combination of violence by the Taliban, ethnic conflict, and natural disasters. Pakistan is also host to one of the largest refugee communities in the world, comprising of Afghan migrants. Displaced people especially in the FATA and KPK provinces have been challenged for many years, with women populations suffering from complex health-related problems. The displaced and refugee women in Pakistan are particularly susceptible to extreme victimization and deprivation, leading to poverty and ill-health (Qayum et al. 2012). Armed conflict and decades of civil war in Sri Lanka have contributed to massive internal displacement. Considerable number of IDPs in the Northern and Eastern provinces of Sri Lanka is a consequence of the 30-year civil war between the government and the Tamil tigers. Violence and abuse against displaced women in Sri Lanka has been extremely high, as women have been purposively used as a war tool for many years to spread fear and force suppression (Kumar 2011).

6.2 Women Households, Work, Ownership, Information Networks, and Poverty

Climate change, conflict, and displacement have combined to cause a chain reaction in male mortality and male migration, leading to an increase in the rate of women-centered households in South Asia (Stapleton et al. 2017). When men of South Asia decide to migrate to earn stable incomes, they leave the women behind to take care of the children, the home, and lands, in an attempt to preserve patriarchal sentiments and safeguard the family honor. Women-centered families waiting for remittances or allowances from migrant male relatives are more likely to have less money and suffer from longer time periods without money all together. This makes them more vulnerable to food insecurity and overall hardships. Though it is well understood that single-women households are commonly impoverished, the conditions of displaced or disaster-affected single-women households is much worse. These households are critically disprivileged groups who lack the resources and knowledge to maintain basic living standards, preventing their potential for bouncing back after disaster. After migration, women on agrarian farms become solely responsible for subsistence farming in order to survive. However, pressure to produce from ravaged and unproductive land impacted by climate change or conflict is extremely difficult and physically strenuous for women, with consequent negative impacts on health and survival of self and children.

Women have always remained the poorer of the two genders (Jerneck 2018). Contexts such as South Asia are additionally marked by limited public investment in strong social security systems, limiting the potential for bouncing back after disaster. Women's risk for deprivation and mortality is considerable when they belong to an unfavorable socioeconomic background, but it is even greater when they experience disasters, conflict, and displacement. Women from lower wealth classes, those who are illiterate or semi-literate, and those who do not work or are employed in the informal sector do not have adaptive capacities to recover from displacement, climate change, and conflict (Aguilar 2009). The age of the women, whether she is currently pregnant, and how many children she has less than the age of 10 years are all factors that would affect the efficiency and health of women when faced with added workloads, caused by displacement and climate change. In addition, the level of education and experience women have has a significant impact on their physical and emotional health while managing additional work from land production or integration in a new region.

As women and girls carry considerable burden for agricultural production and yield across South Asia, any changes in production opportunities due to disaster and conflict impact the livelihood and well-being of women considerably (Rao et al. 2019). Agricultural production by definition is erratic and unpredictable. To compound the predicament, climate change in South Asia is causing higher temperatures which reduces agricultural production and compromises livestock maintenance. The overall work burden for women to manage the home and family and also to produce from the land for family consumption and small incomes multiplies exponentially. As a backup for survival, many women also have to hunt for food in the forest or fish. In addition, the increase in weed and pest proliferation caused by climate change means that women not only suffer due to lesser productivity but increased physical work load for weed and pest control. Land degradation due to climate change requires great investment and capital from affected populations, and most South Asian families, and especially women-centered households, do not have savings or funds for this.

It is the South Asian woman that is more dependent on the natural resources and environment for her livelihood and well-being, as she does not have her educational degree or professional affiliation to fall back on in the event of disaster and need to find new means of revenue. If not agriculture, many South Asian women are employed in fishery, which is being impacted by climate change (Gender and Alliance 2016). Participation in fish processing and trading has been a popular employment option for women who do not have alternatives for home and childcare. As distribution patterns for fish population change due to climate impact, women are left with less fish available for food consumption and employable income. Climate change is also difficult on women whose families are still dependent on patterns of hunting and pastoral activities. Not only is there less to hunt and less water for livestock, but climate change impacts the quality and quantity of gathering food such as berries and fruits, which may be the last recourse for many women to feed their families in the absence of livestock and hunting outcomes. Less options for consumption from fishing and pastoral activities mean less nutrition and health quality of life for women and children.

Many South Asian displaced women are forced to work in the informal sector and in unskilled work due to lack of professional degrees and financial pressures. These informal occupations include home-based work like stitching and embroidery, domestic service like childcare and cleaning, and factory production like textile manufacture. Not only is informal work physically and emotionally draining for displaced women, but it offers limited or no employment benefits and health benefits (Lamb 1996). Women remain deprived of contracts for minimum work hours, leave with pay, maternal benefits, pension, and provident funds; and most importantly, they may be working in hazardous health conditions. As isolated workers and freelance contractors, they may have little bargaining power without organizational assistance on their side. There is little workplace safety or protection for women in unskilled informal work, placing them at risk of exploitation, professional bullying, and sexual harassment. Work in unregulated factories of South Asia which do not have quality measures further exposes women to health hazards such as bad air quality and chemical exposure.

It is argued that resources have to be used efficiently and immediately after disaster or climate change for survival to be achieved (Achieng et al. 2014). As women own less resources and assets to start with, they have less experience with its management and decision-making, thus contributing to why they are weaker partners in development after displacement and climate change. Without resources, capital, land, bank accounts, assets, and professional degrees, women are extremely crippled in resurrecting their lives. South Asian women are known to suffer the systematic disadvantage of being deprived of property and wealth, due to son preference. As daughters, they inherit less land and assets; and as unpaid domestic workers or informal workers, they rarely have the ability to acquire wealth and land. Thus, with lesser ownership of land and assets, women are more vulnerable in the event of disaster and displacement as they are left with fewer buffers such as savings and insurance. South Asian women are also less represented and sponsored by the state, thus receiving less funds and patronage for rehabilitation or land compensation in comparison to men.

Many displaced women, including internal migrants, are without property or assets due to emergency displacement or disasters. There is loss of identity cards and birth certificates and documentation or ownership records which can lead to many bureaucratic hurdles preventing access to health, education, work permits, loan issuance, and other necessities to rebuild lives in displaced communities (Global Protection Cluster Working Group 2007). Eligibility and application for loans, repatriation, and registration can be difficult or delayed, if not impossible, for both genders. Furthermore, success and ease in bureaucratic negotiation and recovery for official documentation and loan issuance in South Asian women are even more problematic due to the complex sociostructural problems, such as limited acceptability and lack of safety for women in bureaucratic offices and exposure and confidence in women themselves.

The structural and social disadvantages faced by women under normal circumstances tend to worsen in times of hardship, uncertainty, and conflict. Women's ability to remain healthy in times of displacement and climate change has also to do irrevocably with their status and privilege across different structures of society, such as the household, community, economy, law and governance. There is a significant role of community norms and values in determining the treatment of women refugees and displaced communities; and additionally, these norms are not consistent across the spaces of South Asia. Whereas men can rely on male networks, kinship, and higher social status, for decisions related to agricultural production and recovery management, women are unable or prevented from using land and resources as effectively (Sraboni et al. 2014). There are multiple stressors for women having to readapt and produce from the land without decision-making ability, which can compound their health issues, including mental health problems. Though microfinance loans have been made available for some women during climate change, South Asian women still do not gain with regard to their health and autonomy, due to dominant utilization of loans by male family members and exclusion of women in decision-making rights (Al-Amin and Chowdhury 2008).

In the age of the information revolution, we assume that all people, including women, have access to information related to health, disaster, or conflict. However, this is not true. Impoverished women and those based in rural and remote locations are known to have less access to digital information, with displaced women ranking last on the list of access to information (Gajjala 2003). Many South Asian women are prevented from accessing local information through the community and marketplace due to restricted mobility. It must also be considered that South Asian women from the urban areas and from the formal working sector also have less time to access general information or health information due to imbalances in home-work equations and lack of assistance for children and domestic responsibilities. It is because of this limited information that women are the last to know about warning signs for disaster or conflict, such as imminent storms or sudden disasters; and they are also less likely to seek early detection or diagnosis for health problems. Women are also less likely to be aware of new immunizations and seasonal risks for infections and thus are less likely to take swift protective measures for health safety of self and child.

Network theory suggests that there are benefits of having weak ties, which allows access to information from distant networks (Granovetter 1983). Men have weak ties as they are more mobile and educated and have been developing a network in the market and at the workplace. The women of South Asia comparatively do not have weak ties, as they communicate and interact with their family, and mostly their children, and they are not exposed to or aware of novel and vital information which may help them in new and unknown circumstances of disaster and conflict. As women do not have access to a distant network, they are unable to benefit from building bridges of information and social capital or make better decisions for displacement recovery and health recovery. In this way, women households of South Asia have greater disadvantages in gains for production, employment, health, and overall survival.

6.3 Shortages of Food and Water, Evacuation Delays, and Life in Displaced Communities

Food insecurity is known to cause comparatively more undernutrition and stunting in girls than in boys, especially during and after displacement, as men and boys are prioritized for food intake in times of shortage (Agarwal and Herring 2013; Iqbal and Amjad 2010). Undernutrition is a major health concern for women, but most especially for displaced women and girls who are suffering physically, growing girls, pregnant and lactating mothers, and victims of violence. Women eat less during times of food shortage primarily because of patriarchy and son preference, but also because social norms and rational choice are used to justify more food for men who are assumed to do more physical tasks and have bigger bodies, thus requiring more food. Physical work for domestic labor, childcare, or reproduction is assumed to not require as much physical strength in regressive South Asian families. Availability of limited supply of livestock and meat for protein consumption is reserved for male members of the family. South Asia also has a history of eliminating and keeping protein and meat diet at a minimum for its women, due to beliefs that it is not necessary for their physical health and that it interferes with their reproductive health. As pressure rises to produce biofuel as a renewable resource from agricultural land, it means more food insecurity for women who have been producing food from limited land (Ahmed and Suphachalasai 2014).

Food insecurity also affects women much more because of intrafamily adaptation to limited food supply, with women themselves choosing to eat less not just due to social conditioning but their own care instinct and protective behavior for family (Alston and Akhter 2016). Displacement and climate change also means that women spend much more time on survival matters, having less time to cook and consume nutritious or adequate meals. Additionally, women may choose or be forced to eat less of the nutritious food and instead fill their stomachs with an unhealthy diet leading to health problems caused by inadequate nutritional levels or overeating of carbohydrates. Even when processed and retail food is available, it is men and boys who have more mobility, access, and finance to consume the extra meals or food that they need. As women are less mobile and culturally restricted to traditional and home-cooked food in South Asia, they face more food deprivation when there is shortage within the household. In some cases, food shortage in displaced communities is being combated with supply of dry rations, which again women and children are more likely to consume due to limited mobility. However, dry food rations are small meal portions which give the illusion of solving food shortages, but instead contribute to health problems like undernutrition, stunting, and starvation in the long run.

The shortage of water caused by climate change, displacement, and having to live in temporary housing as refugees has consequential health consequences on women and the girl child (Rohwerder 2016). One of the main responsibilities of South Asian displaced and climate-affected women include securing water and cooking fuels. Both tasks require strength, time, and energy and are known to impact health and well-being negatively. South Asian women are also less likely to be able to escape from the cycle of ill health caused by sole responsibility to secure and store water and harmful cooking fuels due to cultural barriers for symmetrical household assistance. Water shortages lead to individual-level problems for women such as requiring extra time and energy to collect water from distances and time spent on storing and rationing water in the house. Health-wise this leads to greater physical and emotional burdens on women. On a macro level, water shortages reduce entrepreneurial opportunities and increase poverty levels, contributing to poverty-led ill-health and disease. As a result, women suffer from the health consequences of water shortage more than the men.

Daughters of the house are commonly pulled out of school to assist mothers in collection of water, leading to not just overall reduction in future quality of life of South Asian girls but specific deprivation with regard to health literacy and health awareness. Having to walk long distances and carry heavy storage units for water has physical consequences on bone, joints, and also the growth of young girls. Due to mobility and access restrictions on women, communal tube wells have been developed in some displaced communities of South Asia for water access (Nair 1997). However, arsenic-contaminated wells are known to cause poisoning and related health problems, such as blood in urine, muscle cramps, convulsion, and organ failure leading to death. Other negative consequences of arsenic-contaminated wells include skin pigmentation, skin lesions, and hyperkeratosis which can have mental health effects on women and girls with regard to social acceptability and marriage prospects, but also have general physical effects such as discomfort in daily living due to corns, calluses, or warts.

Women of South Asia have a considerable cultural disadvantage in escaping during climate change and conflict emergencies in comparison to men (Bradshaw and Fordham 2015). South Asian women cannot escape as easily due to less physical mobility, in terms of rigid cultural dress codes such as the sari, shalwar kameez, and burqah, which are not conducive for running, climbing, or swimming. Dress codes for South Asian women also leave them more susceptible to heat waves during climate change, due to excessive and multiple layers of thick cloth. Additionally, women from the region have lack of experience in running and defense due to social barriers and lesser opportunities in school. Training for evacuation and emergencies, and skills in defense are minimalistic for women, and the dilemma is compounded by the fact that women have not been conditioned or trained since childhood to adopt attitudes for emergency responses and defense. The lack of conditioning and training in youth makes it harder for women to learn these skills later in life and especially during times of crisis.

Delayed evacuation of women is a vulnerability which places them at greater risk of adverse health outcomes and also mortality (Economist Intelligence Unit 2014). Women are not only delayed in relocating and escaping, but there are critical consequences to their safety and health due to the delays and the separation of male family guardians when the men leave before them. Women either get left behind, as men are the preferred gender for refugee acceptance, as they can form part of a temporary working population. Evidence shows that many South Asian women are unable to make autonomous decisions for emergency evacuation, due to lack of permission from male relatives, issues of segregation and seclusion in house, and impermissibility for geographical mobility. Lastly, women are also less likely to attempt to escape without their children; and with multiple children and younger children, emergency flight without assistance becomes impossible. Women are also less likely to escape from conflict and disaster situations like entrapment under vehicles or buildings; and they are also less likely to be the ones who are saved or searched for, compared to men and children.

There is clearly only the extreme push factor which drives South Asian women's displacement, as women predominantly from the region would not leave their homes unless there is absolute necessity and life-threatening circumstances (Iqbal and Gusman 2015). It is because of this that South Asian displaced women driven by push factors are extremely vulnerable and defenseless population groups, who are without alternatives and completely dependent on structural and community support for rebuilding of their lives. As it is South Asian women have the highest rates of abuse within the homes, ironically linking domestication and seclusion of women with lack of safety (Niaz 2003). However, displaced women living in refugee camps or temporary housing face even greater risk of abuse, violence, injury, threat, and rape. The risk of sexual harassment and violence is also consequential for girls. If not refugee camps, women displaced populations usually reside in slum areas or temporary housing, where they are also deprived of basic hygienic needs, like clean water, shelter, adequate toilet, and drainage system.

There is little support for the health and autonomy of women and children in these temporary shelters, with critical issues of lack of privacy, holistic healthcare, and lack of opportunities for employment, along with systemic violence and abuse (Donnelly and Muthiah 2017). Refugee shelters that are built without planning and gender sensitivity lack separate or hygienic washing facilities for women, as well as private spaces for bathing, washing, breastfeeding, or changing of menstrual pads (Sang 2018). Many women refuse to evacuate during emergencies caused by climate change due to knowledge that no separate women shelters exist. The state of privacy and permeability of shelters is such that some research suggests that women are forced to use their clothes to construct barriers for privacy. There is also the case of the shelters not providing hygienic environment or privacy for the delivery of child. Women refugees are mostly perceived by host countries or communities as having fewer skills for efficient employability, and thus they are provided less options for paid work, creating more barriers for their health access. Many women in refugee camps have suffered dual problems of stability due to growing hostility and violence from host communities fuelled by delays in resettlement.

Living in displaced communities and refugee shelters has also been evidenced to cause more family level problems for women, leading to both physical and mental health challenges. Abandonment of husbands and estrangement within families is not unknown, with women losing the stability of their family and conjugal bonds (Gomez 2002). In some cases, marital rape has also been reported (Wood 2014). Both climate-affected families and displaced communities in temporary shelters become confined in small spaces; this is especially true for the traditionally controlled women of South Asia. Thus, women of the region face greater risks of infectious diseases. The most common infectious diseases reported in displaced and refugee communities of South Asia are influenza, acute respiratory infections, tuberculosis, malaria, measles, dengue, fever, HIV/ AIDS, Hepatitis B and C, typhoid, and tetanus (John Guzek et al. 2017). Women are more at risk of infectious diseases as they are primary care providers both in the home and at the workplace, and they remain in close proximity within refugee camps or single room households. Women especially restricted by purdah have limited opportunity to remove themselves from within the walls of infection and disease. There is also high risk of vector-borne diseases like malaria and dengue in women, during early morning and evening hours, as most women engage in land management and food or water collection activities in early morning and evening times, when there is less heat and less responsibility for childcare. Women may spend more time near water placing them at risk of water-borne infectious diseases caused by storms and flooding during natural disasters and by standing water in temporary shelters. Women are usually the ones to find themselves immobile and sequestered in flooded regions for prolonged periods due to immobility and having to wait for male members to return after locating migration options or assistance for flood relief. Chronic illnesses like coronary disease, cancer, diabetes, arthritis and other joint problems, kidney failure, and asthma are also a rising concern, with women suffering due to a combination of stress, bad diet, and physical work burdens.

Many girl children living in shelters do not go to school, or attend suboptimal makeshift schools. Their dropout rates are high due to bad quality in the makeshift schools or because they are needed to assist in domestic tasks of the temporary housing (Save the Children Federation 2018). Where camp schools are present, it is the girl child that is known to suffer the most due to abuse and neglect, but also because of rise in political radicalization of boys in schools. The association between lack of schooling and high dropout rates with health literacy and health awareness is momentous and will continue to have negative impact in the long run.

Invariably women living in displaced communities are left without electricity or other power supplies (Lahn and Grafham 2015). This influences the evening study time of girls which requires electricity, as the day is reserved for domestic duties or sibling care for many adolescent girls. Similarly, women who are working from the home and now living in shelters need electricity for home-based production such as sewing machines. For such women, hoping to resume home-based income earning activities, there is little opportunity for small income earning in temporary housing after displacement when they need it most and consequently small income for health and nutrition. The absence of day care for children also reduces ability for women to seek employment outside the shelters. The difficulties of managing psychosocial trauma and not receiving health literacy on how to deal with these problems or skill and development to assume financial autonomy places women and children at life-long risk of lower health quality of life and overall life opportunities.

6.4 Violence, Forced Marriage, Unplanned Pregnancies, and Added Pressure of Care Roles

There is an association between gender-based mortality statistics and displacement; with women and girls more likely to be killed compared to men (OXFAM 2009). Some estimate suggests that mortality after crisis in refugee communities is fifteen times higher than under normal circumstances (John Guzek et al. 2017). The most common reasons for mortality in refugee communities include death due to shooting, physical violence, burning of homes, detention, or kidnapping. For women specifically, there are added difficulties of lower mobility, literacy, and economic empowerment building barriers for them to escape, cope, or survive climate change, conflict, and displacement. Increase in the temperature and extreme heat is also associated with greater mortality in women, due to limited mobility, isolation, and physiological differences.

Gender-based violence against women has a complex intersectionality, with disabled and low status women minorities suffering from greater rates of violence and displaced women suffering even greater rates of violence (Hari 2016). As estimates are not confirmed, it is important to collect data about actual prevalence of different forms of violence that occurs during and after displacement or climate change. Physical and verbal abuse is common, but the risk of sexual threat, rape, and coerced prostitution in vulnerable displaced women and younger girls is extremely high. The neglect of state, laws, and accountability exacerbates women's vulnerabilities in facing violence and abuse from destination communities. Evidence suggests that underage girls are giving birth and becoming mothers after rape victimization, with perpetrators including family members and even fathers (Asnong et al. 2018). There is reason to believe that conflict, displacement, and climate change can lead to extremely deviant and violent behavior in men, who are dealing with crisis and uncertainty by abusing those that they can easily exploit without fearing consequences.

Most importantly, reportage of rape and violence is extremely low, due to fear of backlash or loss of social honor, disabling health and social support for victims and rehabilitation for stability in the future. One of the reasons for low reportage is also because displaced women also face rape and violence at the hands of security personnel, who are meant to be their protectors (Vu et al. 2014). In addition to the physical and mental health consequences of victimization, there is added concern about women's destruction of trust levels and faith in law enforcement and governance permanently. The social-capital theory of health proposes that trust and social cohesion are factors that explain social differences in health. When perpetrators are state and law enforcement agents, there is not just lack of trust and security for women, but it also contributes to building anxiety and stress and weakens her confidence and perceptions of social support. This has consequences for women's ability to rebuild lives in the community, approach the state and legal agents for rehabilitation assistance, and also invest trust in other formal agents like healthcare practitioners.

The dissimilarity-repulsion hypothesis helps to elaborate why women become common targets in displaced communities by reluctant hosts (Chen and Kenrick 2002). Natives perceive dissimilarities based on nationality or ethnicity and thus develop attitudes of dislike against the displaced communities to the extent that they may feel enough revulsion to use violence and abuse. Sometimes anger and resentment against refugee men who are stealing jobs are taken out on the refugee women. Women are not only easy targets, but in South Asia, hurting a woman is equivalent to killing two birds with a stone, as the men are also harmed through their perceptions of family honor. As South Asian women account for the main victims of displacement violence, the long-term ripple effects on mother and child must also be addressed. Children born during and after displacement and children born from rape are part of the next generation who will carry multiple scars of the deprivation and violence of displacement.

It may be argued that displacement is adding to already existing regressive customs against women and girls in South Asia due to multiplying fears and insecurities. The girl child becomes vulnerable to being taken out from school and being forced into marriage as an underage bride or a reluctant one (Myers and Harvey 2011). Forced marriage in times of hardship and insecurity is common in South Asia. Parents of South Asia rely on the custom of dowry to secure financial benefits from their daughters forced or early marriages, and in times of displacement or climate change, poor parents are in extreme need for financial liquidity in order to pay for resettlement and adaptation. Derived from protection motivation theory, it is also true that perhaps child marriages and forced marriages provide vital safety and security for the girl child or young women in a time of uncertainty. Parents and especially elder fathers or single mothers believe that marriage will be a protection against the risk of violence against the girl child and younger women. In this way, more knowledgeable parents who despite knowing the health risks of child marriage may still opt for their underage daughters to be married as they may perceive the health risks of violence and rape to outweigh the health risks of child marriage. Women's self-appraisal of health threat and choices for child marriage of daughters is definitely a coping strategy, but it has multiple and permanent negative health consequences for young girls and any future children they bear.

One may argue that women and girls, who have experienced sexual assault and consequent pregnancies from rape, face the most permanent and damaging physical and mental health problems. Communicable ailments such as dengue, malaria, and cholera are known to be greater risks for pregnant women and the unborn child. The adverse pregnancy risks from floods, heat, violence, stress, and infectious disease include pregnancy complications, miscarriage, premature birth, reduced birth weight, and anemia (Rylander et al. 2013). There is also the risk of emergency deliveries without access to institutions or medical practitioners during times of displacement, conflict, and climate disaster. Finally, there are permanent risks to the unborn child with some research suggesting that extreme weather and violence are a cause for autism, lower intelligence, and lower earnings (Kinney et al. 2008).

South Asian displaced women and girls without protection are at greater risk of illegal trafficking and forced prostitution (Huda 2006). There are layers of health burdens faced by trafficked women including the obvious sexually transmitted diseases, but also the effect on mental health and the sociostructural barriers to accessing healthcare, as such women become ostracized by South Asian communities due to punitive cultures. Illegal professions of sex work may also be voluntary for women who have no environmental security, structural support, or other option to earn an income for themselves and their children. Health risks of prostitution include premature death, sexually transmitted diseases and HIV, drug abuse, accidents, and violence from sexual partners (Sanders 2004). The health risks of prostitution are immense, but they are also consequential when we consider that women may be expecting or lactating. The dangers of fetal alcohol syndrome, related birth defects, and development disabilities are certain, but they are statistically unknown. Mental health problems in women forced into prostitution include depression, posttraumatic stress disorder, and panic disorders. Women are also more susceptible to suicide ideation and morbid thoughts. A large number of such women also become victims of low self-esteem, identity loss, and posttraumatic stress symptoms, all leading to inability to adjust and adapt to change and commit to recovery and rehabilitation.

High rates of drug abuse have also been reported in South Asian displaced women (Horyniak et al. 2016). Substance abuse is primarily embraced by women as a coping strategy to survive loss and manage difficult living conditions or experiences of violence during and after displacement. The health consequences for women after drug use are greater than that in men (Lamy and Thibaut 2010). Harmful metabolites remain in women's bodies longer than in men's, thus increasing comparative health risks of liver, heart, and brain damage, breast cancer, gastric ulcers, and alcoholic hepatitis. In addition, drug abuse can weaken the immune system and cause appetite loss and weight loss, lung damage or failure, mental confusion, strokes, and brain damage. There is also the risk of long-term damage to the body even after substance abuse and the consequences on family. There are great health risks of substance abuse in expectant mothers, lactating mothers, and mothers with younger children exposing their fetus or child to harmful drugs. Children witnessing violence, prostitution, and drug abuse in temporary homes and refugee shelters with little privacy also face substantial risks such as long-term physical and mental health problems, loss of appetite, estrangement from parents and family, adoption of violence and deviant behaviors, and inattention and distraction from school (Hodes 1998).

The natural reproductive role of women must be taken into consideration significantly in regions like South Asia where fertility rates are high. As more women are likely to be pregnant in South Asia, compared to other regions, the health risks to mother and child during climate change and conflict assume greater salience. It is the pregnant woman who has less chance to escape or migrate as easily compared to a nonpregnant woman. Pregnant women are more vulnerable to climate change and displacement mainly due to exposure to excessive heat or infectious diseases, adverse pregnancy risks, and permanent gynecological damage. Global warming is especially risky for pregnant women, as evidence suggests that expectant mothers are more likely to have stillbirths, premature births, or other negative pregnancy outcomes (Poursafa et al. 2015). Women with younger children and pregnant women also suffer from greater stress and anxiety due to compounded uncertainty and insecurity for their children's life prospects and opportunities.

The issue of the safety of the girl child is a momentous concern in displaced communities. Many girls are abducted, sexually abused, and forced to become soldiers to assist rebel or armed forces during conflict (Womens Refugee Commission 2009). Many girl children in South Asia have been impregnated due to rape during and after conflict and displacement. The health consequences of this rape are immense, not to mention the lack of school-related health literacy that these girls will be deprived of due to child pregnancies and motherhood. Child mothers become vulnerable to lifetime suboptimal healthcare practices due to illiteracy and inexperience, and if they survive pregnancy and give birth to a live child, they are less able to secure the health or nutritional needs for their growing child. Expectant mothers forced to give birth in shelters and temporary houses have given birth to stillborn children due to prenatal and pregnancy stress, nutritional deprivation, and physical weakness.

The psychological consequences on the girl child after suffering rape include depression and suicidal tendencies (Bagley et al. 2017). There is also risk that after facing such violence as children they may expect and accept such forms of violence and even become immune to the act and opt for professions of prostitution after being rejected and socially shamed by families. Postnatal depression in child mothers and their means of coping with the burden of a new child have not been researched, but it is obvious that the consequences and impact are devastating. For a region like South Asia, such girls face the prospect of never being able to live fulfilled lives, never being accepted by society, and never having a chance to get married or forget the past. More research is needed about refugee and displaced families who may very well be covertly killing their daughters to save them from violation or abduction, as South Asian families were known to practice this during the years of conflict preceding independence from colonial rule and partition of states in the 1940s.

Many stakeholders and agencies for rehabilitation and resettlement have touted women as change agents, primary facilitators, and saviors (Jerneck 2018). The belief is that women, due to their care ethics and emotional capacity, can be more reliable resources for recovery and adaptation. In this way, women are being held responsible for water management, production on small land holdings, and maintenance of refugee camps. These are additional duties for women, which they have not been socially or physically prepared for, as they are known to be the gender that has received lesser nutrition, educational, and employment opportunities in life. There is no doubt that policy must be designed to support more vulnerable populations like women, children, the elderly, and the disabled during climate change and displacement, but it is not the deprived woman who should be given the burden for relief and adaptation in their micro-habitus. As gender norms and structures stand now, it is ironic that we are asking the oppressed and marginalized women for support in times of critical need. This is almost another form of oppression and exploitation, when women have been afforded lesser resources, capability, and skills to support others while maintaining their own health, both physical and mental.

Social expectations of women exclusively providing emotional labor and care work have created a triple shift burden that has been sustained in South Asia despite modernization. As traditionally perceived care providers, women share the larger burden of care work within the family and in informal work opportunities after displacement. Not only are they responsible for the customary emotional labor of child nurture, adult stabilization, and maintenance of the conjugal, but during and after displacement, they are allocated care work through paid employment opportunities of domestic work and nursemaid duties. There are more sick people to care for during and after climate change, conflict, and displacement, making women informal healthcare providers along with the multiple other care roles they are already expected to perform. Additionally, women are expected to become counselors for children and family members suffering from change, conflict, and displacement, when they themselves are sufferers and victims. The simultaneous and added pressure of having to assume roles as recovery agents in times of displacement and climate change implies a quadruple shift burden on women.

6.5 Mental Health, Health Behavior Patterns, and Health Policy for Displaced Women

As summarized in Table 6.3 and discussed above, there is a web of multiple and intersecting health problems and complications that women face including infectious and noncommunicable diseases, injury and violence, and health issues caused by shortages in food and clean water and lack of permanent or secure housing with basic hygiene facilities. However, less highlighted are the challenges and consequences of mental health issues faced by women affected by climate change, conflict, and displacement. There are substantial psychological consequences in women

Table 6.3 List of environmental alterations faced by women due to displacement and climate change and the corresponding health impacts[a]

Environmental alterations on women caused by displacement and climate change	Subsequent health impact
Increased burden for land produce	Additional physical burden Lack of time for self-health, childcare, nutritious food preparation
Increased burden for income from informal work and unskilled work	Work in factories, farms or homes with no occupational safety Risk of burns Exposure to toxic air or chemicals Poor ventilation and lung disease Low wages and long working hours Violence at hands of employers, co-workers or visitors at workplace
Loss of assets and inability to recover or take loans for asset/ capital build-up	Lack of money for health Mental health burdens Opting for illegal work with health risks
Single-women/ women-only households	Lack of time for self-health, childcare, nutritious food preparation Mental health burdens Poverty-led ill health
Poverty after displacement and climate change	Lack of money for health Mental health burdens Opting for illegal work with health risks
Lack of information networks	Inability to make optimal health decisions or adopt best health behaviors Lack of awareness and knowledge for income generation and
Water shortage	Dehydration Physical burden of carrying water from long distances Diseases born from access to contaminated water or arsenic water Food and income shortage due to less water for agriculture and livestock
Flooding	Infectious diseases Vector-Borne Disease (e.g. dengue and malaria)
Food shortage	Undernutrition and anemia Low birth weight children Starvation and mortality Obesity and diabetes
Heat exposure	Dehydration Weight loss Mortality Slow-down or reduction in daily tasks leading to increased health risks
Air pollution	Respiratory infections Asthma or lung cancer

(continued)

Table 6.3 (continued)

Environmental alterations on women caused by displacement and climate change	Subsequent health impact
Chemical exposure	Weakened immune system and organ damage Allergy and asthma Deformities in fetus and child
Delayed evacuation	Risks in accidents and injuries Physical burden for survival Mental health burden for survival and rescue Greater exposure to infectious diseases
Life in refugee camps and temporary housing or shelters	General exposure to extreme weather Mental health problems (stress, anxiety, depression, suicidal ideation) Risky sexual behavior with spouse or intimate partner Physical and sexual assault Absence of or limited healthcare services in camps Bad quality healthcare services in camps
Violence and abuse	Permanent or temporary physical damage Mental health deterioration Reproductive health complications Pregnancies from rape
Forced marriage, child marriage, and forced prostitution	Physical damage (temporary or permanent) Mental health deterioration Reproductive health complications Pregnancies from rape Sexually transmitted diseases
Pregnancy during displacement, climate change and conflict	Adverse pregnancy risks Greater risk of TB, malaria, HIV Fertility loss or reproductive organ damage
Responsibility for care roles and informal care agents during displacement and conflict	Added care burdens Excessive emotional strain Mental health problems Less time for self-health
General uncertainty and insecurity	Mental health deterioration Obesity and diabetes Undernutrition and anemia Chronic ailments (heart, diabetes, cancer) Drug abuse
Reduced access to reproductive health and family planning	Unplanned pregnancies Adverse pregnancy outcomes
Overall conflict, displacement and climate hazards	Increase in women's mortality Increase in maternal mortality Increase in neo-natal mortality
Lack of citizenship status	No health insurance or coverage No health loans Exclusion from public healthcare services

(continued)

Table 6.3 (continued)

Environmental alterations on women caused by displacement and climate change	Subsequent health impact
Aging population is dominant in displacement	Joint and muscle problems, arthritis and osteoporosis Dementia and Alzheimer's Urinary Incontinence

[a]This table has been compiled by the authors

due to loss of identity and state, financial independence and employment, and home and assets (Delara 2016). Many displaced and refugee populations invariably migrate because they already belonged to unfavorable socioeconomic classes and disprivileged regions. Inequalities and disadvantages are magnified after displacement, causing endless fatigue and hopelessness in women. Women from poor backgrounds with fewer opportunities can become more susceptible to depression, stress, anxiety, and suicide ideation (Silove et al. 2017).

Women, who can have no hope of returning to their old lives, homes, and family, may suffer much more complex and permanent mental health problems. South Asian women also face more psychological abuse from the community and society after climate disasters, conflict, and displacement, compared to the men (Schumacher et al. 2010). This is because the regional culture of South Asia places the blunt of social blame on women in the event of disasters and misfortune. The social expectations are that women through their prayer and piety protect misfortune from harming their homes, family, and children. Similarly, the stigmatization faced by women who are widowed due to disaster and displacement in South Asia is considerable. Widows face considerable social shame and rejection from in-laws and family for having a disadvantaged fate, and they are predominantly shunned from relatives and community, causing even greater mental anguish.

There is the complexity of cyclical ill health in displaced women who incontrovertibly face mental health challenges due to posttraumatic stress but also suffer cyclic highs and lows due to recurring problems of adaptation and resettlement. Transpersonal theory must be considered in context to South Asian displaced women and the influence of healthy ego development on their ability to adapt successfully. As women of the region have been culturally deprived of healthy ego development, through limited opportunities for education and autonomy, which would have built their creativity and knowledge base, they are more prone to psychosis in times of disaster, conflict, and after experiences of violence. This may be why extreme uncertainty for the future and experiences of violence and exclusion have led many displaced women to attempt or commit suicide (Jordans et al. 2014). Women and girls who have been abused are particularly vulnerable, and so women who believe their life chances and opportunities, both economic and social, have been compromised permanently without hope of relief or recovery.

For South Asian women, there is great loss of dignity after displacement as they are conditioned to believe that their social status and honor are linked to the upkeep and stability of their homes and family. With the destruction of home and uprooting of children, women suffer loss in dignity with consequential impact on psychological health. Women forced to remove their face veils by security personnel or parts of their clothing to facilitate escape also suffer loss in dignity. If there is experience of rape and violence against self and daughters, there is high risk of permanent mental health consequences. Many of the women do not face one-off rape and instead suffer from systematic and sustained rape, which has greater physical and mental health consequences (Sang 2018). Women and girls may also suffer greater mental health problems as disaster and uncertainty in a highly conservative region like South Asia drive women's development initiatives further back, especially in the case of education and autonomy. Women of South Asia facing mental health challenges have little cultural support for seeking the help they need, and the lack of available services for mental health support means that the success of readjustment and adaptation is severely compromised.

Health behavior is determined by the socioeconomic background of women including their own literacy and the overall literacy of family members, like parents and spouse (Santow 1995). The household income, family conservatism, healthy literacy, and community acceptability of health access are also factors that influence health behavior of women living in displaced communities. Vulnerable population groups like displaced women and children do not have the finances for out-of-pocket health expenses. Many women living in refugee camps are not allowed to seek healthcare services from male doctors due to cultural constraints and fallacious religious interpretations. Additionally, most women are so focused on survival after displacement and climate change; that health seeking behavior is not a priority for them. The health belief model supports the argument that South Asian displaced women may choose not to actively seek healthcare services due to health illiteracy and perceived lack of benefits, especially in the case of mental healthcare services. Belief codes of South Asian women are developed by cultural constructions of social acceptability, which do not usually include determined or aggressive health-seeking behavior. It would not be wrong to say that some of the debilitating factors behind regressive health behavior in displaced women are because of cultural conditioning and adherence to social norms.

Health behavior and health recovery are invariably related to social support and social integration (Berkman et al. 2000). As women displaced communities are not socially integrated and receive very little social support, their health behavior is severely compromised. There is great discrimination and exclusion in terms of health responsiveness from the host or destination country if they attempt to move away from their camp areas to seek healthcare from centers reserved for regular citizens. Using attachment theory, we may infer that displaced South Asian women who are less secure and attached in the community also face less attachment with healthcare practitioners, health workers, or counsellors. This may be primarily because of experiences of violence and abuse in host country. Further assessment and planning are needed on how to break barriers of approachability and attachment even when health practitioners and providers become available to displaced women. South Asian women follow traditions of seeking community-based healthcare and alternative health services. The transtheoretical model of change is especially applicable to South Asian women, who, after facing violence and displacement, are less willing to allow more changes in their lives by accepting nontraditional healthcare assistance. Providing services to unwilling and reluctant displaced women becomes a further challenge, specifically with regard to assistance for mental health and long-term chronic illnesses.

Five South Asian countries are reported to have the world's greatest number of "new" displacements in 2018, at nearly 3.5 million people (IDMC 2018). These figures suggest that the volume and diversity of displaced people in South Asia is not just great, but it is growing. The major concern is that on-going natural disasters, conflict, and eco-political instability in South Asia have not just kept attention away from the health sector overall but kept women displaced populations invisible. Where health policy is initiated, it is either gender imbalanced or not carried through effectively to make a difference. National adaptation programs that have been initiated have not prescribed any adaptation programs or policies specifically related to the issue of climate displacement (Price 2018). Diligent monitoring of existing and new health services is needed, as evidence suggests that ghost clinics exist without the requisite healthcare practitioners available for assistance in displaced communities (IDMC 2018). Assessment and systematic recording of benefits accrued are also nil, with women satisfaction reports unheard of.

There are immeasurable barriers to accessing healthcare in displaced women communities, including lack of availability, absence of finances, lack of time, and issues of cultural permission to access biomedical healthcare services and services from male healthcare practitioners (Lee et al. 2014; Miller 2018). Though temporary shelters and refugee camps may have provision for primary healthcare services, there is almost no specialized care available at secondary and tertiary level. Those requiring surgical interventions either go without or suffer from risky surgeries, without basic support of general anesthesia, oxygen cylinders, analgesics, and vital surgery-related drugs and equipment. Health manpower and resources are short in all displaced communities, either because displaced communities have been placed in previously empty spaces that did not have health centers or because of overcrowding in established areas (Milton et al. 2017). Healthcare provided by volunteers or semi-trained volunteers can pose a health risk due to lack of training and skill, especially for pregnant women with regard to midwife assistance in camps. Reports by OXFAM confirm that there are no women staff members in refugee planning committees and few women healthcare practitioners in healthcare camps, which is a major barrier to access for conservative South Asian populations. There is further complexity with stateless women not just being the inferior gender but destination governments not wanting to take responsibility for the health sponsorship or health improvement of women refugees, as they are less likely to get absorbed in the informal workforce of the host country (Meyer et al. 2011).

If women are to be nominated as change agents, there needs to be more region-specific assessment for the needs of women in order to facilitate and support their new roles. Critical limitations of South Asian health policies for displaced women include: (i) the estimations of affected women is low and uncertain, thus affecting planning and policy mapping; (ii) there is no formal, consistent, or systematic state support for women; (iii) there is no consideration of differentiation of impact on different women groups; and (iv) there is overdependence on UNHCR and NGOs for relief and recovery of women. The governments of South Asia must come together to do specific and intersectional data collection and policy making with a gender criterion. Collective data collection is vital in order to understand cross-border problems and facilitate reintegration through internal structures and agents. We recommend that the gendered health policy for displaced women communities of South Asia includes the following key areas:

- Systematic and longitudinal collection of health data on women and girl refugees, IDPs and forced migrants, and those affected by climate change. Demographic data must also be collected, such as age, class, ethnicity, provincial belonging, rural belonging, feudal belonging, literacy, occupation, and religious belonging and women headed households. It will then be possible to perform correlation and predictive analysis to assess intersectional predicaments for better policy mapping. Qualitative data collection, like face-to-face interviews and focus group discussions, must also be used to understand specific needs and change in needs and to assess efficacy of health interventions or recommendations by women themselves for needs in health services. Observation methods and ethnographic research are also recommended to continually assess challenges related to abuse and neglect, the interaction of regional political policies, geographical forecasts, and cultural customs on the potency of interventions and policy.
- There is immediate need for women health camps, women health centers, women help desks, women emergency toll numbers, women's health and disease surveillance, and assessment centers. Displaced women must be provided both primary and specialized healthcare services. Special attention needs to be given to reproductive health and even health awareness for birth spacing and family planning through community healthcare workers. Vaccinations and immunizations for displaced mother and children are also needed. Geriatric care for the aging women in displaced communities is also critically required. Mental health counselling services by women counsellors and therapists are also recommended, with sustained therapy and support for victims of violence and sexual assault. The use of women health social workers for counselling, solidarity, and record-keeping is also recommended.
- Improved housing quality, with protection, safety, and privacy, is needed. The introduction of women development officers, women protection officers, and women security in refugee and displaced areas is vital. We also recommend women-only cluster refugee villages to afford safety and privacy. These clusters would help women in water and cooking fuel management activities, collective home-based production for income, and childcare. Within displaced community's development programs for women's health literacy, violence prevention, food and nutrition support, and basic hygiene must be initiated.
- Comprehensive issuance of provisional identification cards across all groups in South Asia is needed. These cards must help women secure loans and ownership

documents without delay. Subsidization to displaced women is necessary, most especially the following subgroups: women headed families, single women, elderly women, disabled women, pregnant and lactating women, girl orphans, and women ethnic/religious minorities. Assistance for loan and grant provision and access to updated information networks are also needed.

- Educational opportunities for girls and younger women, with emphasis on retention in school, are needed, along with segregated schooling. Skill and development training for women to improve employability, especially training in vocational skills, accountancy, and home-based production, is also needed. Occupational and skill flexibility is also a requirement so women can adapt easily for new means of revenues, especially rural and agrarian communities.
- Employee benefits and protection for women working in the informal sector in order to reduce the risks of occupational injury and workplace violence, with health benefits and paid health leave, must become obligatory. Compulsory health insurance must be guaranteed for all displaced populations.

References

Achieng, S., Solomon, A., Cenerini, C., & Di Grazia, A. (2014). *How to deal with people in post-displacement—Reintegration: The welcoming capacity approach*. Rome: Food and Agricultural Organization of United Nations.

Agarwal, B., & Herring, R. (2013). Food security, productivity, and gender inequality. In *The Oxford handbook of food, politics, and society*. New York: Oxford University Press.

Aguilar, L. (2009). Women and climate change: Vulnerabilities and adaptive capacities. *Worldwatch Institute, 59*, 59–62.

Ahmed, M., & Suphachalasai, S. (2014). *Assessing the costs of climate change and adaptation in South Asia*. Philippines: Asian Development Bank.

Al-Amin, M., & Chowdhury, T. (2008). Women, poverty and Empowerment: An investigation into the dark side of Microfinance. *Asian Affairs, 30*, 16–29.

Alston, M., & Akhter, B. (2016). Gender and food security in Bangladesh: The impact of climate change. *Gender, Place & Culture, 23*, 1450–1464.

Asnong, C., Fellmeth, G., Plugge, E., San Wai, N., Pimanpanarak, M., Paw, M. K., Charunwatthana, P., Nosten, F., & Mcgready, R. (2018). Adolescents' perceptions and experiences of pregnancy in refugee and migrant communities on the Thailand-Myanmar border: A qualitative study. *Reproductive Health, 15*, 83.

Bagley, C., Shahnaz, A., & Simkhada, P. (2017). High rates of suicide and violence in the lives of girls and young women in Bangladesh: Issues for feminist intervention. *Social Sciences, 6*, 140.

Berkman, L. F., Glass, T., Brissette, I., & Seeman, T. E. (2000). From social integration to health: Durkheim in the new millennium. *Social Science & Medicine, 51*, 843–857.

Bradshaw, S., & Fordham, M. (2015). Double disaster: Disaster through a gender lens. In *Hazards, risks and disasters in society*. Amsterdam: Elsevier.

Chen, F. F., & Kenrick, D. T. (2002). Repulsion or attraction? Group membership and assumed attitude similarity. *Journal of Personality and Social Psychology, 83*, 111.

Chhabra, S. (2018). Effects of Societal/Domestic Violence on Health of Women. *Journal of Women's Health and Reproductive Medicine, 2*(1), 6.

Delara, M. (2016). Social determinants of immigrant women's mental health. *Advances in Public Health, 2016*, 1–11.

Donnelly, E. R., & Muthiah, V. (2017). *Protecting women and girls in refugee camps*. Center for Women, Peace and Security, London School of Economics, London, UK.

Economist Intelligence Unit. (2014). *The South Asia women's resilience index: Examining the role of women in preparing for and recovering from disasters*. London: The Economist.

Gajjala, R. (2003). South Asian digital diasporas and cyberfeminist webs: Negotiating globalization, nation, gender and information technology design. *Contemporary South Asia, 12*, 41–56.

Gender, G., & Alliance, C. (2016). *Gender and climate change: A closer look at existing evidence*. Global Gender and Climate Alliance: New York.

Global Protection Cluster Working Group. (2007). *Handbook for the protection of internally displaced persons*. Global Protection Cluster Working Group.

Gomez, M. (2002). National Human Rights Commissions and Internally Displaced Persons. *Illustrated by the Sri Lankan Experience An Occasional Paper July The Brookings–SAIS Project on Internal Displacement*.

Granovetter, M. (1983). *The strength of weak ties: A network theory revisited*. San Francisco: Jossey-Bass.

Hari, K. (2016). Disability discourse in South Asia and global disability governance. *Canadian Journal of Disability Studies, 5*, 25–62.

Härkönen, M. (2016). *Tibetan Nuns between Oppression and Opportunities: An Intersectional Study*. Helsinki: University of Helsinki.

Hasan, M., Sutradhar, I., Shahabuddin, A., & Sarker, M. (2017). Double burden of malnutrition among Bangladeshi women: A Literature review. *Cureus, 9*, e1986.

Hasan-ul-Bari, S., & Ahmed, T. (2018). Ensuring sexual and reproductive health and rights of Rohingya women and girls. *The Lancet, 392*, 2439–2440.

Hodes, M. (1998). Refugee children: May need a lot of psychiatric help. *British Medical Journal Publishing Group, 316*(7134), 793–794.

Horyniak, D., Melo, J. S., Farrell, R. M., Ojeda, V. D., & Strathdee, S. A. (2016). Epidemiology of substance use among forced migrants: A global systematic review. *PLoS One, 11*, e0159134.

Huda, S. (2006). Sex trafficking in South Asia. *International Journal of Gynecology & Obstetrics, 94*, 374–381.

IDMC. (2018). *Global Report on Internal Displacement*. Geneva: Internal Displacement Monitoring Centre (IDMC).

Iqbal, M., & Amjad, R. (2010). Food security in South Asia: Strategies and programmes for regional collaboration. In *Regional integration and economic development in South Asia* (Vol. 357). Cheltenham: Edward Elgar.

Iqbal, M., & Gusman, Y. (2015). Pull and Push Factors of Indonesian women migrant workers from Indramayu (West Java) to work abroad. *Mediterranean Journal of Social Sciences, 6*, 167.

Jerneck, A. (2018). What about gender in climate change? Twelve feminist lessons from development. *Sustainability, 10*, 627.

John Guzek et al. (2017). Health Survey in Kutupalong and Balukhali Refugee Settlements, Cox's Bazar, Bangladesh. Medecins Sans Frontieres Survey Report. https://www.msf.org/sites/msf.org/files/coxsbazar_healthsurveyreport_dec2017_final1.pdf

Jordans, M. J., Kaufman, A., Brenman, N. F., Adhikari, R. P., Luitel, N. P., Tol, W. A., & Komproe, I. (2014). Suicide in South Asia: A scoping review. *BMC Psychiatry, 14*, 358.

Khatiwada, P. P., & Bakhundol, L. (2010). *Conflict induced migration in Nepal* (a social inclusion perspective). PhD Unpublished, Tribhuvan University, Kathmandu.

Kinney, D. K., Miller, A. M., Crowley, D. J., Huang, E., & Gerber, E. (2008). Autism prevalence following prenatal exposure to hurricanes and tropical storms in Louisiana. *Journal of Autism and Developmental Disorders, 38*, 481–488.

Kumar, S. (2011). Conflict and internal displacement in Sri Lanka: Concerns and obstacles to durable solutions. In *Finding a point of return: Internally displaced persons in Sri Lanka* (pp. 1–10). Kolkatta: Mahanirban Culcutta Research Group.

Lahn, G., & Grafham, O. (2015). *Heat, light and power for refugees. Saving lives, reducing costs*. London: Royal Institute of International Affairs.

Lamb, C. (1996). *Barriers to work for refugee women*. Second women in migration conference.
Lamy, S., & Thibaut, F. (2010). Psychoactive substance use during pregnancy: A review. *L'Encephale, 36*, 33–38.
Lee, S. K., Sulaiman-Hill, C. R., & Thompson, S. C. (2014). Overcoming language barriers in community-based research with refugee and migrant populations: Options for using bilingual workers. *BMC International Health and Human Rights, 14*, 11.
Marbach, M. (2018). On imputing UNHCR data. *Research & Politics, 5*, 2053168018803239.
Meyer, S., Tappis, H., Weiss, W., Spiegel, P., & Vu, A. (2011). Refugee site health service utilization: More needs to be done. *American Journal of Disaster Medicine, 6*, 231–242.
Miller, S. D. (2018). *Assessing the impacts of hosting refugees*. Waterloo: Centre for International Governance Innovation.
Milton, A., Rahman, M., Hussain, S., Jindal, C., Choudhury, S., Akter, S., Ferdousi, S., Mouly, T., Hall, J., & Efird, J. (2017). Trapped in statelessness: Rohingya refugees in Bangladesh. *International Journal of Environmental Research and Public Health, 14*, 942.
Myers, J., & Harvey, R. (2011). *Breaking vows: Early and forced marriage and girls' education*. Report prepared by: Plan- Because I am a Girl, London. UK. https://plan-uk.org/file/breaking-vows-efm-3462225pdf/download?token=RlE5iobL
Nair, R. (1997). Refugee Protection in South Asia. *Journal of International Affairs*, 201–220.
Niaz, U. (2003). Violence against women in South Asian countries. *Archives of women's mental health, 6*, 173–184.
OXFAM (2009). Fact sheet climate change & women, OXFAM America. https://s3.amazonaws.com/oxfam-us/www/static/oa3/files/climatechangewomenfactsheet.pdf
Poursafa, P., Keikha, M., & Kelishadi, R. (2015). Systematic review on adverse birth outcomes of climate change. *Journal of Research in medical Sciences: The Official Journal of Isfahan University of Medical Sciences, 20*, 397.
Preet, R., Nilsson, M., Schumann, B., & Evengård, B. (2010). The gender perspective in climate change and global health. *Global Health Action, 3*, 5720.
Price, R. A. (2018). *Women-initiated measures to cope with environmental stresses and climate change in South Asia* (K4D Helpdesk report). Brighton: Institute of Development Studies.
Qayum, M., Mohmand, S., & Arooj, H. (2012). Frequency and physical factors associated with gender-based violence in the internally displaced people of Pakistan. *Journal of the College of Physicians and Surgeons Pakistan, 22*, 63–65.
Rao, N., Gazdar, H., Chanchani, D., & Ibrahim, M. (2019). Women's agricultural work and nutrition in South Asia: From pathways to a cross-disciplinary, grounded analytical framework. *Food Policy, 82*, 50–62.
Rohwerder, B. (2016). *Women and girls in forced and protracted displacement*. Birmingham: Governance and Social Development Resource Center.
Roshan, B. (2004). The more things change, the more they stay the same: The plight of Afghan women two years after the overthrow of the Taliban. *HeinOnline*.
Rylander, C., Øyvind Odland, J., & Manning Sandanger, T. (2013). Climate change and the potential effects on maternal and pregnancy outcomes: An assessment of the most vulnerable–the mother, fetus, and newborn child. *Global Health Action, 6*, 19538.
Sanders, T. (2004). A continuum of risk? The management of health, physical and emotional risks by female sex workers. *Sociology of Health & Illness, 26*, 557–574.
Sang, D. (2018). *One Year On: Time to put women and girls at heart of the Rohingya response*.
Santow, G. (1995). Social roles and physical health: The case of female disadvantage in poor countries. *Social Science & Medicine, 40*, 147–161.
Save the Children Federation, I. (2018). *Hear it from the Teachers- Getting refugee children back to learning*, Save the Children USA. https://resourcecentre.savethechildren.net/node/14237/pdf/hear-it-from-the-teachers-refugee-education-report.pdf
Schumacher, J. A., Coffey, S. F., Norris, F. H., Tracy, M., Clements, K., & Galea, S. (2010). Intimate partner violence and Hurricane Katrina: Predictors and associated mental health outcomes. *Violence and Victims, 25*, 588.

Silove, D., Ventevogel, P., & Rees, S. (2017). The contemporary refugee crisis: An overview of mental health challenges. *World Psychiatry, 16*, 130–139.

Sraboni, E., Malapit, H. J., Quisumbing, A. R., & Ahmed, A. U. (2014). Women's empowerment in agriculture: What role for food security in Bangladesh? *World Development, 61*, 11–52.

Stapleton, S. O., Nadin, R., Watson, C., & Kellett, J. (2017). *Climate change, migration and displacement: The need for a risk-informed and coherent approach*. London: Overseas Development Institute.

UN Population Division. (2017). *International migrant stock: The 2017 revision*. United Nations Department of Economic and Social Affairs-Population Division.

UNHCR. (2018). *Mid year trends 2018*. UNHCR The UN Refugee Agency.

United Nations Development Programme. (2009). *Human Development Report 2009- Overcoming barriers: Human mobility and development*. New York: United Nations.

Vu, A., Adam, A., Wirtz, A., Pham, K., Rubenstein, L., Glass, N., Beyrer, C., & Singh, S. (2014). The prevalence of sexual violence among female refugees in complex humanitarian emergencies: A systematic review and meta-analysis. *PLOS Currents Disasters*. pp 1–19. Edition 1. https://doi.org/10.1371/currents.dis.835f10778fd80ae031aac12d3b533ca7

WHO South-East Asia Region. (2018). *Health of refugees and migrants*, WHO South-East Asia Region Report. https://www.who.int/migrants/publications/SEAROreport.pdf?ua=1

Womens Refugee Commission. (2009). *Refugee Girls: The Invisible Faces of War*. New York: Womens Refugee Commission.

Wood, E. J. (2014). Conflict-related sexual violence and the policy implications of recent research. *International Review of the Red Cross, 96*, 457–478.

Chapter 7
Social Barriers to Mental Well-Being in Women of South Asia

Masha Asad Khan, Sara Rizvi Jafree, and Tahira Jibeen

7.1 Introduction

Mental distress refers to psychological disorders which effects changes in cognition, emotions, and behavior, resulting in disabled function within the family, society, and work (Galderisi et al. 2015). Under the broad umbrella of mental health distress, three hundred specific disorders have been defined. Latest calculations from the World Health Organization (WHO) in 2015 indicate that over 300 million people experience depression globally and approximately 264 million people are suffering from anxiety disorders worldwide. Globally, mental distress in women is higher compared to men, and women between the ages of 15 and 44 years are at greater risk (Thara and Patel 1998). Estimates exert that by 2020 depression will become the second most cardinal contributor of mental health disorders among women (Murray and Lopez 1996; Trivedi et al. 2007).

Around two billion people live in the South Asian region, with 48% of the population consisting of women. Women of South Asia are known to commonly face problems related to domestic violence, gender inequity, and sexual abuse, placing them at greater risk for mental health challenges (Jacob et al. 1998). The common mental health challenges among South Asian women include: (i) post-traumatic stress disorder, (ii) dissociative disorders, (iii) conversion and depression, (iv) self-harm and suicide, and (v) eating disorders (Akol et al. 2018). Several problems with

M. A. Khan (✉)
Applied Psychology Department, Kinnaird University, Lahore, Pakistan

S. R. Jafree
Department of Sociology, Forman Christian College University, Lahore, Pakistan

T. Jibeen
Advance Health, Toronto, Canada

ClinicVillage Centre, Mississauga, Canada

S. R. Jafree (ed.), *The Sociology of South Asian Women's Health*,
https://doi.org/10.1007/978-3-030-50204-1_7

defining mental health and reporting it are also found in South Asian women, such as: (i) believing that reporting mental health problems is equivalent to reporting a personal weakness and (ii) confusion between mental health and decision-making or governance autonomy (Aziz et al. 2011). To add to the problem, there are excessive cultural barriers in South Asia preventing women from talking about their mental health and seeking healthcare (Trivedi et al. 2007). Shame and guilt are used as strategies within the family to discourage talk of mental distress. It is known that when individuals suffer in silence with constant feelings of hopelessness and despair, it not only aggravates mental health problems but can also lead to physical symptoms, like chronic pain and digestive difficulties (World Health Organization 2015).

Many argue that patriarchal oppression is responsible for leaving a lethal impact on South Asian women's psychological well-being (Reddy and Chandrasekhar 1998; Trivedi et al. 2007). South Asian communities have still not recovered from rigid gender stereotyping which contributes to mental distress in girls and women (Burr 2002). There is also the role of class, with some women from the upper classes able to access healthcare from private practitioners and lower-class women remaining deprived due to public healthcare shortfalls. Traditional beliefs that women with mental health challenges are possessed by evil spirits or are victims of black magic still persist in contemporary days (Gies-Powroznik 2016). Due to these regressive beliefs, many women in South Asia suffer from grave social ostracization and family neglect (Banu 2016). Women sufferers can face abandonment at the hands of their family, society, and government, leaving them deprived of basic shelter, food, and clothing.

There is also the grave issue of criminality being attributed to mentally ill women in South Asian communities. Poor women in the region who face serious mental health challenges without early care have been known to end up in mental asylums (Niaz and Hassan 2006). Women in asylums have been fed stale food and rendered with inappropriate seasonal clothes (Chesler 2005; Somasundaram and Ratnaraj 2018). Furthermore, treatment approaches in asylums for "mad" or "insane" women consist mostly of moral therapies rather than medication and therapy (Pinto 2014). Such abandoned and institutionalized women also suffer from greater risks of physical, verbal, and sexual abuse (Calabrese and Dorji 2014).

7.2 Social Risk Factors for Mental Distress in South Asian Women

There is need to create awareness in the South Asia region regarding mental distress and to highlight the fact that it is a consequence of socio-cultural factors (Yu 2018). In this part of the chapter, we will discuss the main socio-cultural predictors of mental health challenges faced by women of the region. Women belonging to South Asian communities come from collectivist setups and consequently develop their sense of self through the roles and worth assigned to them through family (Lefley 1987). A salient historical discrimination that assails South Asian society is the desire and expectation of a male child, which is still prevalent in contemporary times. A female child is never "wanted" and her birth is reluctantly accepted as an unfortunate event, with major blame placed on the mother. This forms the foundation of low self-esteem, personality problems, and weak sense of self-worth in daughters and mothers of South Asia (Szymanski and Henning 2007). A very important psychological factor that perpetuates mental distress symptoms and hinders the South Asian woman from seeking professional help is the absence of self-compassion (Neff 2003).

Perpetual fears of endangering family honor in a collectivist society deepens women's mental distress and psychological comorbidities (Naved et al. 2006). There is thus the dilemma of underreporting in South Asia, as women are conditioned not to disclose mental distress. Rastogi et al. (2014) carried out a study with clinicians who provided care to South Asian clients with mental health issues. It was reported that women sufferers who managed to secure a psychotherapist came accompanied by male relatives, mostly their husbands. The male companions answered for the women and strongly dominated the reporting of clinical case and treatment plans. Many women suffering from mental distress were forced to drop out of therapy because their male relatives did not believe in the treatment plan and thus refused to pay for the treatment. The patriarchal belief being that help-seeking behavior for mental distress in women is unnecessary and a "Western" practice (Dein and Sembhi 2001; Razali et al. 1996). Milder versions of anxiety and depression in women to this day are "normalized" and attributed to personality weakness. More commonly women are advised to seek family ties and religious rituals rather than counseling or professional therapy (Romans and Seemans 2013; Khan et al. 2015). Ultimately, South Asian women living in a patriarchal setup are unable to benefit from a support network for mental healthcare services (Romans and Seemans 2013).

Lack of social support and regressive customs related to coming of age for girls and menstruation in South Asia also has an important relationship with mental health. "*Gupha basne*" is a custom in some Hindu Nepali communities that means "staying in a cave." Women who menstruate are made to stay in a darkened room for up to 12 days. A similar tradition that breaches basic human rights exists in Nepal and is known as "*chhaupadi*," by which women are made to live alone in huts away from their homes during menstruation (Ranabhat et al. 2015). Many women are forbidden to share a bed with their husband, enter the kitchen, touch food or food utensils, or touch their father or brother during menstruation (Crawford et al. 2014). Social exclusion and shaming related to menstruation can significantly affect daily activities, mental well-being, and social life in girls and women (Mouli and Patel 2017). Healthcare workers in South Asia have not developed protocols to support the psychological challenges caused by cultural treatment of menstruation (Nillni et al. 2011).

A cultural belief held among South Asian communities till today is that marriage and motherhood can substantially reduce mental distress and curtail certain "evil" symptoms such as depression and emotional instability (Sharma et al. 2013). However, scholarship suggests that support from husbands and in-laws is not always favorable for women of the region (Qadir et al. 2013; Dommaraju and Jones 2011). Wives who suffer from preexisting mental health disorders may face mistrust and abuse by husband and in-laws (Srivastava 2013) and consequently face emotional and physical abuse, psychological distancing, and incompatibility problems (Behere et al. 2011). From another perspective, it is also true that many South Asian women suffer from mental distress after marriage due to cultural customs such as normalization of intimate partner violence and acceptance of second marriages. Not only do South Asian women victims of intimate partner violence underreport physical injuries, but they also ignore the mental distress associated with experiences of spousal violence (Jejeebhoy et al. 2014).

Traditional practices like exchange marriage or watta satta are also known to contribute to high risk for abuse and mental health deterioration in women of the region (Niaz 2004). Another regressive practice associated with marriage is the dowry system, which is known to have a negative impact on women's mental health and self-worth (Huda 2006). Absence of dowry or unsatisfactory dowry size can lead to marital discord, maltreatment, and domestic violence, which have been found to be major psychological stressors for women (Ali et al. 2013). South Asian literature is also indicative of increased psychiatric morbidity after the birth of a child. Many cultural factors are known to contribute to postnatal depression such as fatigue, birth of a girl child, and lack of assistance in childcare (Howard et al. 2013). Cyclical poverty and dysfunctional family system can also cause higher prevalence of certain mental distresses like postpartum depression (Fisher et al. 2012). Finally, widowed and divorced women have low social acceptance and face great stigmatization in the region, and they consequently are known to experience higher rates of mental health problems (Trivedi et al. 2009).

Zafar and Malik (2016) investigated the decision-making power for women's reproductive health and found that even literate and urban-dwelling women faced mental distress due to low decision-making power. Women had to seek permission to go out of the homes for routine grocery shopping and even emergency checkups at hospitals. Even if working women had autonomy to seek healthcare, the final decision of choosing which doctor they went to was made by the family and mother-in-law. Nonworking women had no participation in decision-making from conception to the choice of a gynecologist. As nonworking women are financially dependent on their husband or male relatives, they remained submissive despite dissatisfaction, leading to adverse mental well-being (Sahithya and Reddy 2018). Nonworking women are particularly affected by orthodox beliefs regarding the prohibition of family planning. It is believed that a woman's dishonor is equivalent to dishonoring the entire family, with the burden of keeping that honor intact placed on the shoulders of male family members. As disclosure about mental health problems in women is perceived as a loss of family honor, many male relatives seek clandestine services from unlicensed faith healers for their women in the country (Saeed et al. 2000).

With rising numbers of special needs children, almost 15% of children in South Asia, we must consider the mental health of mothers with special needs children. It is not uncommon to hear of the mother facing blame and physical abuse when she bears a disabled child, as children are culturally considered to be an investment for the future (Divan et al. 2012). The mothers of special needs children undergo life-long stress which disturbs their marital life, maternal role, and work participation. Research has found a higher rate of parental divorce or marital discord among parents of a child with disabilities compared to parents who have healthy children (Risdal and Singer 2004). Absence of psychosocial support for mothers causes great isolation and guilt, leading to maternal depression (Ilias et al. 2018). Additionally, mothers of special needs children are known to internalize their own health problems and ignore their mental distress in order to selflessly provide care for children who are socially stigmatized and structurally neglected in South Asia (Qasim et al. 2015).

Mothers of special needs children also have to undergo excruciating stress during and after the diagnosis, due to lack of social support by family members, relatives, and society (Khan et al. 2013). A research conducted in Pakistan reviewed the awareness level and beliefs regarding autism from psychiatrists, speech therapists, occupational therapists, physicians, clinical psychologists, pediatricians, and child neurologists (Imran et al. 2011). Results revealed delays and complications during diagnosis and inadequate healthcare system and structural support for the disabled, which added to the emotional strain in mothers (Daley 2004). Majority of husbands in the region are reluctant to pay for the treatment of special needs children, including costs for medication and therapy, which contributes to mental health deterioration in mothers (Ahmed et al. 2016).

The role of religion in sustaining mental health problems is substantial in South Asia, as the region is ruled by conservative forces that interpret religion usually to the detriment of women's health. Many South Asian families believe that mental distress is caused by the "evil eye" and that prayer and piety are enough defenses as a cure (Dein et al. 2008). Classic Muslim ascription for mental distress in South Asian women includes demonic possession, penalty for past sins, or spiritual detachment from God (Salib and Youakim 2001; Kianpoor and Rhoades 2006). Schemas of the modern Indian women can psychoanalytically be understood through popular culture that unconsciously pushes women to be like Sita, the ideal woman in Hindu mythology. The ideal of womanhood incorporated by Sita is one of chastity, gentleness, and acceptance of domestic violence (Kakar 1978). Consequently not only are Hindu women discouraged from sharing their problems and any mental distress, but they are also shamed in the name of religion for showing any weaknesses and mental distress.

As many South Asians believe that mental health disorders and depression can be cured through stronger beliefs and observing religious rituals, this burden is also beared by women (Cinnirella and Loewenthal 1999). Women in religiously conservative societies suffering from mental distress are criticized for their lack of piety and spirituality (Koenig 2012). They are advised to combat their anxiety and depression with religiosity and faith, which can complicate their mental health condition further (Chadda and Deb 2013; Gailits et al. 2019). Faith healers and religious clerics are preferred to mental health practitioners as the former are considered to have greater spiritual power, while the latter are seen with mistrust, thus aggravating treatment and recovery in suffering women (Walaa and Vohra 2013; Inayat 2007).

7.3 Socioeconomic Costs of Neglecting Women's Mental Health

Research on women's mental health usually concentrates on the individual costs and rarely assesses the impact on the society and economy. Neglecting women's mental health has serious and reverberating effects on wider society and can cause permanent damage within the family social order (World Health Organization 2000). The children of mothers with mental distress are at risk for multiple problems including neglect by mother, having to assume household responsibilities for mother, and in extreme cases the loss of mother. Research suggests that children of clinically depressed mothers are at higher risk for mental distress themselves and may have problems related to family function and adult development (Kohl et al. 2011). In addition, children with distressed mothers are known to have lower academic results and less adaptability and suffer from greater conflict and instability. As a consequence, neglecting the mental health of mothers can increase the challenges and costs of the health and education ministries and the economy overall. Specifically, more concentrated efforts would be needed for child health and child monitoring, special education services, and crime management in society.

The major burden of care provision within South Asian families, for both children and the elderly, lies on the shoulders of women (Ferrant et al. 2014). As the primary care providers in the house, women of the region have little time for their own health needs. A research conducted by Rodrigo et al. (2013), on caregiver strain, revealed that nearly half of the women caregivers for sufferers with schizophrenia and bipolar disorder needed professional mental help themselves (Rodrigo et al. 2013). It is not uncommon for caregivers for mentally distressed sufferers to experience mental health deterioration. Women care providers also suffer from physical abuse at the hands of their patients, which exacerbates their emotional strain and mental stability. Women care providers often have to leave their jobs as they are unable to fulfill their professional roles, and the consequent loss of income and autonomy is also known to contribute to mental distress (Pradeep et al. 2018).

Ignorance and neglect of mental health needs of women results in lower productivity and earning potential for the economy. In addition, a number of antisocial behaviors such as homelessness, increased crime rates, drug use, alcohol dependency, and domestic violence are found to be associated with women's mental health distress, which have their own socioeconomic costs respectively (Rueve and Welton 2008). Bloom et al. (2014) estimate that fiscally India is at a risk of losing USD 1.03 trillion, before 2030, due to adverse mental health challenges. Health costs are also compounded when mental health is not diagnosed correctly or timely. Some mental health issues are not considered serious in South Asia like eating disorders (Wales et al. 2017). Inadequate and unfavorable quality of services for mental health contributes to increase in suffering and multiple morbidities in women. Rahman (2007) sheds light on how simple depression if not treated can convert into multiple health problems like diabetes and heart disease.

Generally a woman's decision to seek help is the amalgamated result of quality of services provided by the health sector, such as: (i) availability of mental healthcare providers; (ii) feasible location of therapists and costs of transport; (iii) private practice of psychologists, consultancy fee, and cost of antipsychotics or therapy; and (iv) availability of women therapist or counselor. Hospitals with psychiatric wards in South Asia are rare and if found are located only in urban areas or metropolitan cities (Thara and Padmavati 2013). The scarcity of mental health practitioners such as psychologists, nurses, and community health workers in ratio to the women population are also salient structural constraints for health seeking behavior in South Asian women (Khan et al. 2015). Finally, a combination of local problems, such as regional instability and economic insecurity, prevents women from seeking early help for mental health, which can compound health problems and lead to aggravated health costs for the economies of South Asia.

7.4 Country-Specific Analysis for South Asia

In this section of the chapter we will be taking a look at the mental health of women from specific South Asian states including Bangladesh, India, Nepal, Pakistan, and Sri Lanka. From secondary data that is available for South Asia at country level, we can assess the prevalence of mental health problems. However, we must consider the problem of underreporting and that statistics must be read with caution. In Table 7.1 we have presented country-wise mental health disorder prevalence percentages in South Asia. We find that in all five countries mental health disorder prevalence is higher in women than in men [in 2017, women compared to men suffer greater mental health disorders by: 1.7% in Bangladesh, 0.1% in India, 0.5% in Nepal, 0.9% in Pakistan, and 0.2% in Sri Lanka]. We have discussed earlier in this chapter how patriarchal, traditional, and cultural forces in South Asia have led to women suffering greater mental health problems compared to men. With regard to specific mental health disorders, women suffer greater incidence, compared to men, of: (i) anxiety, (ii) depression, (iii) bipolar disorder, and (iv) eating disorders. Over a period of 5 years, from 2012 to 2017, incidence of mental health disorders in women was relatively the same.

In Table 7.2 we present mental and substance use disorder rates, suicide rates, and DALYs (disability-adjusted life years) for countries of South Asia. We find that in all five countries, mental and substance use disorder rate for 2017 ranges between minimum 10,936.5 (Sri Lanka) and maximum 14,257.5 (India) per 100,000 people. This is extremely high and in absolute numbers converts to considerable millions of people in the region. Suicide rates are high and for 2017 they range between minimum 6.0 (Bangladesh) and maximum 19.8 (Sri Lanka) per 100,000 people. DALYs

Table 7.1 Country-wise mental health disorder prevalence percentages in South Asia

	Bangladesh				India				Nepal				Pakistan				Sri Lanka			
	2012		2017		2012		2017		2012		2017		2012		2017		2012		2017	
	W	M	W	M	W	M	W	M	W	M	W	M	W	M	W	M	W	M	W	M
Mental health disorder prevalence	13.6	11.8	13.3	11.6	14.6	14.5	14.6	14.5	13.3	12.7	13.0	12.5	12.5	11.7	12.4	11.5	12.5	12.2	12.4	12.2
Prevalence of anxiety disorders	5.2	3.3	5.2	3.3	3.9	2.7	3.9	2.7	4.6	3.0	4.6	3.1	4.6	3.1	4.6	3.1	4.2	2.4	4.2	2.5
Prevalence of bipolar disorder	0.6	0.6	0.6	0.6	0.6	0.6	0.6	0.6	0.6	0.6	0.6	0.6	0.6	0.6	0.6	0.6	0.6	0.5	0.6	0.5
Prevalence of depression	5.3	3.1	5.1	3.1	4.1	2.9	4.1	2.9	4.4	3.0	4.2	2.9	4.3	2.4	4.3	2.4	3.8	3.1	3.8	3.1
Prevalence of eating disorders	0.2	0.1	0.2	0.1	0.2	0.1	0.2	0.1	0.2	0.1	0.2	0.1	0.2	0.1	0.2	0.1	0.2	0.1	0.2	0.1
Prevalence of schizophrenia	0.2	0.3	0.2	0.3	0.2	0.3	0.2	0.3	0.2	0.3	0.2	0.3	0.2	0.3	0.2	0.3	0.2	0.3	0.2	0.3

Source: This data has been retrieved from publically available data by 'Our World in Data',: https://ourworldindata.org/mental-health

Table 7.2 Mental and substance use disorder rates, suicide rates, and DALYSs (disability-adjusted life years) for South Asia, both genders

	Bangladesh		India		Nepal		Pakistan		Sri Lanka	
	2012	2017	2012	2017	2012	2017	2012	2017	2012	2017
Mental and substance use disorder rate, per 100,000	12,429.5	12,204.4	14,357.4	14,257.5	12,774.8	12,472.2	11,749.8	11,622.4	11,135.1	10,936.5
Suicide rate, per 100,000	6.7	6.0	17.0	15.6	8.7	8.4	4.7	4.5	21.0	19.8
DALYs for mental and substance use disorders	5.0%	5.7%	4.1%	4.7%	4.7%	5.0%	3.0%	3.5%	6.1%	6.3%

Source: This data has been retrieved from publically available data by 'Our World in Data': https://ourworldindata.org/mental-health

for mental and substance use disorders for 2017 are also high with percentages ranging from minimum 3.5% (Pakistan) to maximum 6.3% (Sri Lanka).

Research from Bangladesh shows a high prevalence of lifetime physical and emotional spousal violence against women (Johnston and Naved 2008). Naved and Akhtar (2008) found that spousal violence was linked to suicidal ideation in Bangladeshi ever married women. Islam et al. (2018) found that women facing emotional and verbal violence were at higher risk for conversion disorders, bipolar mood disorders, obsessive compulsive disorders, and acute stress disorders. Most of the abused women, in urban and rural areas of Bangladesh, remain silent about their experience and do not seek healthcare (Parvin et al. 2016). The main reasons for women's silence include fears of: (i) endangering family honor, (ii) tarnishing their own reputation, (iii) jeopardizing their child's future, and (iv) abandonment or violence by husband. Many women in the country also believe that discussing mental health with practitioners will not benefit them, as their problems are caused by rigid socio-cultural norms (Hassan and Thornicroft 2018).

Women in Bangladesh are also more likely to have staunch beliefs in Jinn possession and evil eye and their first priority for management and therapy of mental distress is a religious authority (Mullick et al. 2013). Triggers for anxiety and depressive symptoms in Bangladeshi women are known to be associated with the quality of the relationship with intimate partners, such as: violence, polygamy, and lack of general support (Edhborg et al. 2015). Findings from villages in Bangladesh reveal that mental health counseling along with active community participation can reduce the incidence of intimate partner violence and mental health problems (Schuler and Nazneen 2018). Families in Bangladesh have been facing the agonizing effects of natural disasters on mental health since the 1970s (Nahar et al. 2014). Women are more likely to be affected by the impact of natural disasters as they have restricted physical mobility and cultural barriers to rehabilitation. They are consequently known to suffer from post-traumatic stress disorder, depression, or anxiety following cyclones and disasters. Even after natural disasters women survivors have the demanding duty of household management and recovery in the absence of utensils and assets that have been lost in the disaster. Other reasons women are more vulnerable to psychological distress post-disaster are due to exposure to sexual harassment, poverty, and loss of male family members (Islam et al. 2018).

A preview of the current status mental health development in India tells that health models and mental health acts have been devised but are deficient in implementation. Implications of the Mental Healthcare Act 2017 on women could be better if there is execution and enforcement of its provisions subject to budgetary support (Kaur 2017). Mostly people of the region perceive mental distress to be caused by supernatural causes such as: (i) breach of taboos, (ii) black magic, (iii) evil eye, or (iv) wrath of a god/goddess (Ferngren 2014). The status of mental healthcare for women in India is largely dependent on the use of Ayurveda (Banerjee 2008). Ayurveda is still perceived as a balanced medicine system especially for women, whereas Western medicine is perceived as having negative side effects. This is a perception that is shared by not only uneducated or semiliterate village women in the country but also the educated and professional urban classes.

Ayurvedic medicines are considered neutral, whereas antipsychotic medication is often believed to have an intense heating effect on the gut. Hence, women with mental health problems are reluctant to follow a psychiatric treatment plan.

Media content reveals deep-rooted patriarchal philosophies of male dominance, with women seldom shown in empowering roles and equal relationships (Pandve and Banerjee 2007; Swaminath and Bhide 2009). Ramasubramanian and Oliver (2007) also identified that violence against women was normalized, thus reinforcing such behavior in male members of society. This may be why significant numbers of women in India face domestic violence, leading to high risk for depression, mental distress, and even suicide (Davar 1995). Researchers found that grassroots workers have to make at least five home visits before a domestic violence survivor can be motivated to join therapy or visit the nearest counseling service point (Bhat et al. 2007). Chakraborty (1990) found that Indian women particularly belonging to low- or middle-level professions reported high stress as compared to their male colleagues. Moreover, women in unspecified work groups like beggars, sex workers, and housekeeping maids reported high rates of mental distresses.

Nepal does not have a national mental health program and the limited mental health services currently being provided in the country are due to NGOs (Regmi et al. 2004). Only 0.08% of the health budget is spent on mental health and much of the services are not availed by women due to the conservative culture. Suicide and mental health problems are the lead cause of death in women of reproductive age group in the country (Simkhada et al. 2015). Socio-cultural factors contributing to this high incidence of suicide and mental health disorders include marital violence and marital conflict and expectations of submission to men. Studies have also highlighted high rates of self-harm in Nepalese women who are unable to escape their life circumstances or gain approval from demanding families (Subba et al. 2009). Other literature suggests that women living in traditional family structures and those suffering from husband's alcoholism and polygamy are at high risk for depression (Dorheim Ho-Yen et al. 2007). There is critical need for preventive and curative healthcare services in the country, which is only possible through government investment.

An analysis of Pakistan's mental health system for women shows: (i) inefficient resource allocation and inadequate primary healthcare integration (Hussain et al. 2018), (ii) lack of political commitment (Nishter 2004), and (iii) the absence of trained practitioners for the diagnosis, treatment, and referral of mental health conditions (Malik and Khan 2016). General physicians in the Pakistani medical setup have often been accused of misleading mentally distressed clients because they are not well-versed in the field of psychology. Among prominent structural barriers, sociopolitical instability, war-related violence, economic struggles, and natural disasters, multiple women in Pakistan are plagued with mental health challenges (Mubbashar and Saeed 2002). Gender bias in mobility and negative labels related to women's use of traditional healers lead to differences in seeking help and therapy. Muslim clients in Pakistan initially resort to sorcery, Sufism, Naturopathy (tibb), and multiple folk medicinal treatment methods (Farooqi 2006). The male adult sufferers make more visits to male healers than the women because of the patriarchal system and the conservative restrictions on women mobility. Before approaching psychiatrists, majority of the sufferers including women have sought some form of traditional healing for somatic symptom disorder, anxiety, affective disorders, and personality disorders.

According to a report by the WHO, only 0.4% of the total budget is allocated to mental healthcare in Pakistan (World Health Organization 2015). A further challenge for policy-makers is that with underreporting of mental health problems, there is inadequate planning and budgeting. A cross-sectional survey in the twin metropolitan cities of Rawalpindi and Islamabad in northern Pakistan revealed some ground realities of the current mental healthcare scenario in terms of gender inequality (Qadir et al. 2013). The finding was that daughters, who face discrimination from parents due to their gender, internalize this prejudice by wanting their first child to be a boy. Such women who have gender-based prejudices and son preference are at high risks for psychological morbidity in the country. The fear is that gender-based inequality is internalized by women and then transmitted to the next generation of daughters in a never-ending cycle sustaining mental distress and emotional instability.

Sri Lanka has a pluralistic mental health system with a complex interplay of indigenous, Ayurvedic, and Western models being used simultaneously (Minas et al. 2017). Sri Lankan women have limited social space in which they can have cathartic meetings with other women to discuss gender-related issues (Guzder 2011). Mental health stigma in the country further hinders their willingness to seek professional help. Women in the country have been found to be at high risk of mental health problems when their partners consume alcohol and when they face domestic violence (Hussein 2005). It is because of this that the Ministry of Health in Sri Lanka decentralized mental healthcare and depends on over 80 volunteer organizations to provide mental healthcare to women at community level (Fernando et al. 2017).

Sri Lanka is known to be the suicide capital of the world and second only to China (Vijayakumar 2004). In 2006, alarming rates were recorded in the rural areas with predominant incidences occurring in adolescent girls due to: (i) domination and abuse by male relatives, (ii) extreme poverty and employment problems, and (iii) dysfunctional family systems. Scholarship claims that women in the country commit suicide to draw attention to the wrongs that community and family have imposed upon them (Marecek 2006). The programs currently running in Sri Lanka are limited to mental healthcare for women living in urban areas and majority of the psychiatrists in the country are practicing in the three largest cities (Mental Health Directorate 2015). This indicates that there is a critical treatment gap between rural and urban areas when it comes to the mental health needs of women.

7.5 Case Study: Thematic Analysis of the Perceptions of Women Primary Healthcare Physicians Regarding Mental Health of South Asian Women

Primary care physicians face the complex challenge of dealing with both medical and mental illness. At the same time primary care physicians are the most suitable healthcare practitioners for timely detection and early care of mental distress in women. South Asian women primary care practitioners have unique knowledge about the mental health problems of their own women, due the conservative climate and preference for female practitioners for women patients. A total of 30 women primary healthcare physicians from Pakistan, India, Bangladesh, Sri Lanka, and Nepal were interviewed through phone and email in 2019 by the authors and their research assistants. Ethics approval for this study was taken from Forman Christian College, University, Internal Review Board. Participants were recruited through establishing contact through social media groups on Facebook.

All women participants were current practitioners and empirical evidence of rising mental health problems in South Asian women was shared with them as part of the information cover letter for the study. Two broad questions were asked of participants: (1) their experience of coexistence of mental health problems and medical problems and (2) social and structural barriers to mental healthcare services. All the women practitioners indicated that the mental healthcare services in their respective countries were not satisfactory and that reportage by women was not satisfactory due to a punitive and blame culture. The findings were summarized into broad categories and subcategories as presented in Table 7.3.

We found that women who suffer from mental health problems also suffer from the following medical conditions: (i) chronic disease burden, (ii) reproductive burdens, (iii) physical immobility due to disease and pain, (iv) nutritional problems, (v) victimization from violence, (vi) suffering due to role burden, and (vii) other health issues like vitamin D deficiency and postmenopausal syndromes. We do not know if these medical conditions are predictors of mental health problems, but there may be high likelihood. A more robust study would be needed to prove this. We also found that the following socio-structural barriers prevent adequate mental healthcare services from reaching South Asian women, including: (i) measurement and prevalence problems, (ii) awareness and definition issues, (iii) poverty and prioritization for physical health, (iv) inadequate healthcare services, (v) government shortfalls, and (vi) necessity of integrating major predictors (such as maternal healthcare, food security, education and employment, and regressive traditions perpetuating gender-based inequalities). Our case study results suggest that the use of primary physicians in mental health services and support for women in the communities is imperative in South Asia. With the training and integration of primary care physicians for mental health services at grassroots and community levels, there would be improved detection, early care, and referral system for women of South Asia.

Table 7.3 Findings for coexistence of mental health and medical problems and socio-structural barriers to improved healthcare, as perceived by practicing women primary healthcare physicians of South Asia[a]

Area	Category	Subcategories
Medical problems coexisting with mental health problems	Chronic disease burden	Breast cancer Ovarian cancer Diabetes
	Reproductive burden	Infertility Birth of daughter(s) Multiple pregnancies without gaps Polycystic ovary syndrome
	Physical immobility due to disease and pain	Osteoporosis Arthritis
	Nutritional problems	Undernutrition and food shortage Obesity
	Victim of violence	Verbal abuse Physical abuse Rape
	Suffering from role burden	Heavy workload and burnout due to paid work Asymmetrical burden for domestic work, child care, and care for dependents at home
	Other health issues	Vitamin D deficiency Postmenopausal syndromes
Social and structural barriers to improved women's mental healthcare	Measurement and prevalence	Precise data for prevalence Longitudinal assessment Lack of reporting
	Awareness and definition	Shame associated with mental health distress Punitive culture which blames the sufferer Religious misinterpretation Defining and identifying different types of mental health conditions
	Poverty	Lack of finances for mental health services Prioritization of health costs favoring physical health problems
	Inadequate healthcare services	No or inadequate ward and consultants in both public and private sector hospitals Shortage of trained psychiatrists Lack of training of primary physicians Absence of mandatory screening at primary level

(continued)

Table 7.3 (continued)

Area	Category	Subcategories
	Government shortfalls	Low budget allocation for mental healthcare Inadequate healthcare policy and planning at federal and provincial level
	Necessity of integrating major predictors	The need to integrate mental healthcare with maternal healthcare Ensuring nutritional awareness and food security Improving education and employment Improving regressive traditions: child marriage and inheritance deprivation

[a]Data in this table has been compiled by the authors

7.6 Concluding Recommendations

We can conclude from this chapter that the mental health of South Asian women is adversely affected by socio-cultural factors, such as: (i) lack of awareness and distorted social constructions of mental distress, (ii) patriarchal values and traditionally regressive culture, (iii) marriage expectations and fertility burdens, and (iv) religious fallacies. We may conclude the need to transform mental healthcare support for South Asian women by keeping socio-cultural factors at the forefront while formulating advanced training programs. In addition, there are considerable barriers to accessing mental healthcare services due to: (i) poverty and prioritization or saving of health finances for physical health, (ii) preference for folk medicine and traditional healers, and (iii) major public and private sector shortfalls. We further conclude that there needs to be greater focus on improving awareness and mental health services.

The gap that initially existed in South Asia for women's mental healthcare has widened due to growing mental health challenges and due to regional and economic pressures and increasing population rates (Samy et al. 2015). Where health policy for mental health has been devised, implementation has been weak across the region. We thus recommend strong adoption by the federal and provincial governments for extensive integration of mental healthcare services. This is possible when policy-makers and governments of South Asia commit to an increase in budget allocation, staffing, and resources for mental healthcare services. There is dire need for training of specialists through public financing mechanisms and the introduction of nonspecialist psychosocial support provided through networks of community members at primary level (The National Health Policy 2017). Policy-makers, therapists, and mental health practitioners collectively need to address some barriers that hinder care for mental health problems experienced by South Asian women.

There are considerable women in mental distress in the region who need immediate support or relief from their social conditions and family arrangements (Sahithya and Reddy 2018). For such women we recommend daycare centers, halfway homes, sheltered workshops, and temporary-stay facilities across both rural and urban areas. As South Asia is currently dominated by NGO services for mental health, we also recommend formal monitoring for the function and efficacy of NGO mental health programs for women (Hussain et al. 2018). However, for the long run research highlights that women would sustainably gain mental relief when stigma against mental health is reduced and women are empowered through systematic government schemes, media literacy, and small participatory programs (Schuler et al. 2013). Collective mental health services run by government and private providers, psychology personnel, and social workers are needed to support women for therapy and integration. The main focus for mental health services should be to enable the poor, rural, and marginalized women to retain their dignity and independence so they can lead a productive life (Rastogi and Therly 2006). Overall, South Asian women's mental health problems will also improve once gender equality indicators of educational access, employment opportunities, and social status improve.

A successful mental healthcare system for women in South Asia needs extensive efforts by stakeholders. As South Asia is influenced by religious values, there needs to be more integration of religious psychology in therapy and counseling interventions. Counseling for Indian women can include the fundamental importance of the concept of *Shakti*, meaning spiritual feminine power or energy which is held closely by Hindu women. This can serve as a route to transform the therapeutic process (Sharma and Slate 2013). For Muslim communities awareness and support though religious leaders and local Imams is recommended. Formal training and licensing of faith healers as well as homeopaths is also critical. Hall and Livingston (2006) recommended that therapists form an alliance with the Islamic clergy to clarify Muslim norms and worldview about distress and health, facilitation of referrals, and effective application of treatment strategies. Investment in such endeavors is crucial for the adoption and success of mental health services in South Asia (Ali et al. 2013).

In this contemporary world with social media and technological domination, there are also substantial opportunities for spreading awareness and improving cultural support for women with mental distress (Naved et al. 2006). Many support groups are already available through the Internet for mental well-being, especially for women who are: (i) suffering from postpartum depression, (ii) experiencing infertility problems, and (iii) providing care for special needs children. The further utilization of digital technology to influence access to qualified psychiatrists through the Internet and mobile-based services is a possibility (Sahithya and Reddy 2018). For South Asian women living in remote locations suffering from access issues and those who have social mobility restrictions, e-counseling can become an important option for services. Basic psychological consultation through the Internet can also become home-based career options for many women in the region.

Access to mental healthcare is not homogeneous across South Asia, with service availability strikingly worse in rural parts compared to urban areas. An average South Asian woman's decision to engage with a particular mental health counseling or therapy service is affected by a range of socioeconomic factors such as age and literacy, wealth class and social position, the type of distress or disorder, access to clinics or practitioners, and perceived quality of the mental health service (Tipping and Segall 1995). Pragmatic action plans are needed in South Asian underdeveloped communities to identify perception biases, create awareness of basic mental health rights, and eradicate barriers for help-seeking behaviors. There is empirical evidence that community-based interventions combining women and men benefit women in terms of improved social support, knowledge of rights, and mental health support (Naved et al. 2018). Group therapy, focusing on consciousness raising, needs to be provided to men specifically in order to improve support for women's mental healthcare. To combat sustained patriarchy in the region we propose that preventive awareness should focus on male privilege, male-perpetrated violence, and the "price of masculinity," which often becomes one of the major root causes of mental distress for women of South Asia (Levant and Pollack 1995).

References

Ahmed, S., Ali, J., & Sanauddin, N. (2016). Patriarchy in family care-giving: Experiences of families of children with intellectual disability in Pakistan. *Journal of Postgraduate Medical Institute (Peshawar-Pakistan), 30*(1).

Akol, A., Moland, K. M., Babirye, J. N., & Engebretsen, I. M. S. (2018). "We are like co-wives": Traditional healers' views on collaborating with the formal child and adolescent mental health system in Uganda. *BMC Health Services Research, 18*(1), 258. https://doi.org/10.1186/s12913-018-3063-4.

Ali, T. S., Arnadottir, G., & Kulane, A. (2013). Dowry practices and their negative consequences from a female perspective in Karachi, Pakistan- a qualtiative study. *Health, 5*(7D), 84–91.

Aziz, A., Shams, M., & Khan, K. S. (2011). Participatory action research as the approach for women's empowerment. *Action Research, 9*(3), 303–323.

Banerjee, M. (2008). Ayurveda in modern India: Standardization and pharmaceuticalization. In D. Wujastyk & F. M. Smith (Eds.), *Modern and global Ayurveda: Pluralism and paradigms* (pp. 201–214). New York: State University of New York Press.

Banu, A. (2016). *Human development, disparity and vulnerability: Women in South Asia* (UNDP Human Development Report pp. 3–10). Retrieved: http://hdr.undp.org/sites/default/files/latest_edited_banu_template_gl_1_august.pdf

Behere, P. B., Rao, S. T., & Verma, K. (2011). Effect of marriage on pre-existing psychoses. *Indian Journal of Psychiatry, 53*(4), 287–288. https://doi.org/10.4103/0019-5545.91900.

Bhat, R., Maheshwari, S. K., Rao, K., & Bakshi, R. (2007). *Psychosocial aspects of marital disharmony in mental health care pilots in Gujarat. Processes, outcomes and learning*. Ahmedabad, India: Indian Institute of Management.

Bloom, D. E., Cafiero-Fonseca, E. T., Candeias, V., Adashi, E., Bloom, L., Gurfein, L., & Saxena, A. (2014). *Economics of non-communicable diseases in India: The costs and returns on investment of interventions to promote healthy living and prevent, treat, and manage NCDs*. Geneva: World Economic Forum.

Burr, J. (2002). Cultural stereotypes of women from South Asian communities: Mental health care professionals' explanations for patterns of suicide and depression. *Social Science and Medicine, 55*(22), 835–845.

Calabrese, J. D., & Dorji, C. (2014). *Traditional and modern understandings of mental distress in Bhutan: Preserving the benefits of each to support gross national happiness*. Retrieved from http://www.bhutanstudies.org.bt/publicationFiles/JBS/JBS_Vol30/v30-1.pdf

Chadda, R. K., & Deb, K. S. (2013). Indian family systems, collectivistic society and psychotherapy. *Indian Journal of Psychiatry, 55*(2), 299–309. https://doi.org/10.4103/0019-5545.105555.
Chakraborty, A. (1990). *Social stress and mental health: A social psychiatric field study of Calcutta*. New Dehli: Sage.
Chesler, P. (2005). *Women and madness: Epidemiology and its limits*. Garden City: Doubleday.
Cinnirella, M., & Loewenthal, K. M. (1999). Religious and ethnic group influences on beliefs about mental distress: A qualitative interview study. *British Journal of Medical Psychology, 72*(4), 505–524.
Crawford, M., Menger, L., & Kaufman, M. (2014). 'This is a natural process': Managing menstrual stigma in Nepal. *Culture, Health & Sexuality: An International Journal for Research, Intervention and Care, 16*(4), 426–439.
Daley, T. C. (2004). From symptom recognition to diagnosis: Children with autism in urban India. *Social Science & Medicine, 58*(7), 1323–1335.
Davar, B. (1995). Mental distress among Indian women. *Economic and Political Weekly, 30*(45), 2879–2886.
Dein, S., & Sembhi, S. (2001). The use of traditional healing in south asian psychiatric patients in the U.K.: Interactions between professional and folk psychiatries. *Transcultural Psychiatry, 38*(2), 243–257. https://doi.org/10.1177/136346150103800207.
Dein, S., Alexander, M., & Napier, A. D. (2008). Jinn, psychiatry and contested notions of misfortune among East London Bangladeshis. *Transcultural Psychiatry, 35*(1), 31–55.
Divan, G., Vajaratkar, V., Desai, M. U., Strik-Lievers, L., & Patel, V. (2012). Challenges, coping strategies, and unmet needs of families with a child with autism spectrum disorder in Goa. *India Autism Research, 5*, 190–200.
Dommaraju, P., & Jones, G. (2011). Divorce trends in Asia. *Asian Journal of Social Science, 39*(6), 725–750.
Dorheim Ho-Yen, S. I. G. N. E., Tschudi Bondevik, G., Eberhard-Gran, M. A. L. I. N., & Bjorvatn, B. (2007). Factors associated with depressive symptoms among postnatal women in Nepal. *Acta Obstetricia et Gynecologica Scandinavica, 86*(3), 291–297.
Edhborg, M., Nasreen, H., & Kabir, Z. N. (2015). "I can't stop worrying about everything"-Experiences of rural Bangladeshi women during the first postpartum months. *International Journal of Qualitative Studies for Health and Well Being, 10*, 26226.
Farooqi, Y. N. (2006). Traditional healing practices sought by muslim psychiatric patients in Lahore, Pakistan. *International Journal of Disability, Development and Education, 53*(4), 401–415.
Fernando, N., Suveendran, T., & Silva, C. D. (2017). Decentralizing provision of mental health care in Sri Lanka. *WHO South-East Asia Journal of Public Health, 6*(1), 18–21.
Ferngren, G. B. (2014). *Medicine and religion: A historical introduction*. Baltimore: Johns Hopkins University Press.
Ferrant, G., Pesando, L. M., & Nowacka, K. (2014). *Unpaid Care Work: The missing link in the analysis of gender gaps in labour outcomes*. Issues paper.
Fisher, J., Cabral de Mello, M., Patel, V., Rahman, A., Tran, T., Holton, S., & Holmes, W. (2012). Prevalence and determinants of common perinatal mental disorders in women in low- and lower-middle-income countries: A systematic review. *Bulletin of the World Health Organization, 90*(2), 139–149.
Gailits, N., Mathias, K., Nouvet, E., Pillai, P., & Schwartz, L. (2019). Women's freedom of movement and participation in psychosocial support groups: Qualitative study in northern India. *BMC Public Health, 19*(1), 725. https://doi.org/10.1186/s12889-019-7019-3.
Galderisi, S., Heinz, A., Kastrup, M., Beezhold, J., & Sartorius, N. (2015). Toward a new definition of mental health. *World Psychiatry, 14*(2), 231–233.
Gies-Powroznik, N. (2016). *Madness and mental health in South Asian settings*. Working papers in social anthropology (No. 3). Institute of Ethnology.
Guzder, J. (2011). Women who jump into wells: Reflections on suicidality in women from conflict regions of the Indian subcontinent. *Transcultural Psychiatry, 48*(5), 585–603.

Hall, R. E., & Livingston, J. N. (2006). Mental health practice with Arab families: Implications of spirituality vis-a-vis Islam. *The American Journal of Family Therapy, 34*, 139–150.
Hassan, M. T., & Thornicroft, G. (2018). Mass media campaigns to reduce mental health stigma in Bangladesh. *Lancet Psychiciatry, 5*(8), 616.
Howard, L. M., Oram, S., Galley, H., Trevillion, K., & Feder, G. (2013). Domestic violence and perinatal mental disorders: A systematic review and meta-analysis. *PLoS Medicine, 10*(5), e1001452. https://doi.org/10.1371/journal.pmed.1001452.
Huda, S. (2006). Dowry in Bangladesh: Compromizing women's rights. *South Asia Research, 26*(3), 249–268.
Hussain, S., Khan, M., Gul, R., & Asad, N. (2018). Integration of mental health into primary healthcare: Perceptions of stake holders. *East Mediterranean Health Journal, 24*(2), 146–153.
Hussein, A. (2005). *Sometimes there is no blood: Domestic violence and rape in rural Sri Lanka.* Colombo: International Centre for Ethnic Studies.
Ilias, K., Cornish, K., Kummar, A. S., Park, M. S., & Golden, K. J. (2018). Parenting stress and resilience in parents of children with autism spectrum disorder (asd) in southeast asia: A systematic review. *Frontiers in Psychology, 9*, 280. https://doi.org/10.3389/fpsyg.2018.00280.
Imran, N., Chaudry, M. R., Azeem, M. W., Bhatti, M. R., Choudhary, Z. I., & Cheema, M. A. (2011). A survey of autism knowledge and attitudes among the healthcare professionals in Lahore, Pakistan. *BMC Pediatrics, 11*, 107. https://doi.org/10.1186/1471-2431-11-107.
Inayat, Q. (2007). Islamophobia and therapeutic dialogue: Some reflections. *Counseling Psychology Quarterly, 20*, 287–293. https://doi.org/10.1080/09515070701567804.
Islam, M. M., Jahan, N., & Hossain, M. D. (2018). Violence against women and mental disorder: A qualitative study in Bangladesh. *Tropical Medicine and Health, 46*, 5. https://doi.org/10.1186/s41182-018-0085-x.
Jacob, K. S., Bhugra, D., Lloyd, K. R., & Mann, A. H. (1998). Common mental disorders, explanatory models and consultation behavior among Indian women living in the UK. *Journal of Royal Society of Medicine, 91*(2), 66–71.
Jejeebhoy, S. J., Santhya, K. G., & Acharya, R. (2014). Violence against women in South Asia: The need for the active engagement of the health sector. *Global Public Health, 9*(6), 678–690.
Johnston, H. B., & Naved, R. T. (2008). Spousal violence in Bangladesh: A call for a public-health response. *Journal of Health, Population, & Nutrition, 26*(3), 366–377.
Kakar, S. (1978). *The inner world: A psycho-analytic study of childhood and society in India.* Delhi: Oxford University Press.
Kaur, K. (2017). Implications of the mental healthcare act 2017 on the rights of women with mental distresses in India. *Journal of International Women's Studies, 19*(4), 3–14.
Khan, M. A., Siddique, N., & Jibeen, T. (2013). A comparative study of adjustment problems among mothers of autism spectrum disorder and normal children. *Pakistan Journal of Professional Psychology: Research and Practice, 4*, 1–11. ISSN-1818-6416.
Khan, K. S., Rafique, G., Bawani, S. A., Hasan, F., & Haroon, A. (2015). Social and societal context of women's mental health, what women want, what they get: Gap analysis in Pakistan of mental health services. Policies and research. In N. Khanlou & F. B. Pilkington (Eds.), *Women's mental health, resistance and resilience in community and society* (pp. 33–50). Cham/Heidelberg: Springer International Publishing.
Kianpoor, M., & Rhoades, G. F. (2006). Djinnati, a possession state in baloochistan. *Iranian Journal of Trauma Practice, 4*(1–2), 147–155.
Koenig, H. G. (2012). *Religion, spirituality, and health: The research and clinical implications.* Retrieved from https://www.hindawi.com/journals/isrn/2012/278730/
Kohl, P. L., Jonson-Reidd, M., & Drake, B. (2011). Maternal mental distress and the safety and stability of maltreated children. *Child Abuse Neglect, 35*(5), 309–318.
Lefley, H. P. (1987). Impact of mental distress in families of mental health professionals. *Journal of Nervous and Mental Disease, 175*, 613–619.
Levant, R. F., & Pollack, W. S. (1995). *A new psychology of men.* New York: Basic Books.

Malik, M. A., & Khan, M. M. (2016). Economic burden of mental distresses in Pakistan. *Journal of Mental Health Policy and Economics, 19*(3), 155–166.
Marecek, J. (2006). Young women's suicide in Sri Lanka: Cultural, ecological and psychological factors. *Asian Journal of Counseling, 13*(1), 63–92.
Mental Health Directorate. (2015). *The mental health policy of Sri Lanka: 2005–2015*. Colombo: Ministry of Heathcare and Nutrition.
Minas, I., Mendis, J., & Hall, T. (2017). Mental health system development in Sri Lanka. *Mental Health in Asia and the Pacific Historical and Cultural Perspectives, 1*.
Mouli, V. C., & Patel, S. V. (2017). Mapping the knowledge and understanding of menarche, menstrual hygiene and menstrual health among adolescent girls in low- and middle-income countries. *Reproductive Health, 14*(30), 12–16.
Mubbashar, M. H., & Saeed, K. (2002). Developing models of balanced mental health care: The case of Pakistan. *World Psychiatry, 1*(2), 100–101.
Mullick, M. S., Khalifa, N., Nahar, J. S., & Walker, D.-M. (2013). Beliefs about jinn, black magic and evil eye in Bangladesh: The effects of gender and level of education. *Mental Health, Religion & Culture, 16*(7), 719–729.
Murray, J. L., & Lopez, A. D. (1996). *The global burden of disease: A comprehensive assessment of mortality and disability from diseases, injuries and risk factors in 1990 and projected to 2020. Harvard School of Public Health*. Boston: World Health Organization.
Nahar, N., Blomstedt, Y., Wu, B., Kandarina, I., Trisnantoro, L., & Kinsman, J. (2014). Increasing the provision of mental health care for vulnerable, disaster-affected people in Bangladesh. *BMC Public Health, 14*, 708. https://doi.org/10.1186/1471-2458-14-708.
National Health Policy. (2017). Retrieved https://mohfw.gov.in/sites/default/files/9147562941489753121.pdf
Naved, R. T., & Akhtar, N. (2008). Spousal violence against women and suicidal ideation in Bangladesh. *Women's Health Issues, 18*(6), 442–452.
Naved, R. T., Azim, S., Bhuiya, A., & Perrson, L. A. (2006). Physical violence by husbands: Magnitude, disclosure and help-seeking behavior of women in Bangladesh. *Social Science & Medicine, 62*, 2917–2929.
Naved, R. T., Mamun, M. A., Mourin, S. A., & Parvin, K. (2018). A cluster randomized controlled trial to assess the impact of SAFE on spousal violence against women and girls in slums of Dhaka, Bangladesh. *PLoS One, 13*(6), e0198926. https://doi.org/10.1371/journal.pone.0198926.
Neff, K. (2003). Self-compassion: An alternative conceptualization of a healthy attitude toward oneself. *Self and Identity, 2*, 85–102.
Niaz, U. (2004). Women's mental health in Pakistan. *World Psychiatry, 3*(1), 60.
Niaz, U., & Hassan, S. (2006). Culture and mental health of women in South-East Asia. *World Psychiatry: Official Journal of the World Psychiatric Association, 5*(2), 118–120.
Nillni, Y. I., Toufexis, D. J., & Rohan, K. J. (2011). Anxiety sensitivity, the menstrual cycle, and panic disorder: A putative neuroendocrine and psychological interaction. *Clinical Psychology Review, 31*(7), 1183–1191. https://doi.org/10.1016/j.cpr.2011.07.006.
Nishter, S. (2004). Prevention of non-communicable diseases in Pakistan: An integrated partnership-based model. *Health Research Policy and Systems, 2*, 7.
Pandve, H., & Banerjee, A. (2007). Do popular media such as movies aggravate the stigma of mental disorders? *Indian Journal of Psychiatry, 49*(2), 144. https://doi.org/10.4103/0019-5545.33267.
Parvin, K., Sultana, N., & Naved, R. T. (2016). Disclosure and help seeking behavior of women exposed to physical spousal violence in Dhaka slums. *BMC Public Health, 16*, 383. https://doi.org/10.1186/s12889-016-3060-7.
Pinto, S. (2014). *Daughters of Parvati: Women and madness in contemporary India*. Philadelphia: University of Pennsylvania Press.
Pradeep, B. S., Gururaj, G., Varghese, M., Benegal, V., Rao, G. N., Sukumar, G. M., ... & Bhaskarapillai, B. (2018). National mental health survey of India, 2016-rationale, design and methods. *PLoS One, 13*(10), e0205096.

Qadir, F., Khalid, A., Haqqani, S., Huma, Z., & Medhin, G. (2013). The association of marital relationship and perceived social support with mental health of women in Pakistan. *BMC Public Health, 13*, 1150. (2013). https://doi.org/10.1186/1471-2458-13-1150.

Qasim, N., Mehboob, S., Akram, Z., & Masrour, H. (2015). Women's liberation: The effects of patriarchal oppression on women's mind. *International Journal of Asian Social Science*, 382–393.

Rahman, A. (2007). Challenges and opportunities in developing a psychological intervention for perinatal depression in rural Pakistan–a multi-method study. *Archives of Women's Mental Health, 10*(5), 211–219. https://doi.org/10.1007/s00737-007-0193-9.

Ramasubramanian, S., & Oliver, M. B. (2007). Activating and suppressing hostile and benevolent racism: Evidence for comparative media stereotyping. *Media Psychology, 9*(3), 623–646.

Ranabhat, C., Kim, C. B., Choi, E. H., Aryal, A., Park, M. B., & Doh, Y. A. (2015). Chhaupadi culture and reproductive health of women in Nepal. *Asia Pacific Journal of Public Health, 27*(7), 785–795.

Rastogi, M., & Therly, P. (2006). Dowry and its link to violence against women in feminist psychological perspectives. *Trauma, Violence and Abuse, 7*, 66–77.

Rastogi, P., Khushalani, S., Dhawan, S., Goga, J., Hemanth, N., Kosi, R., et al. (2014). Understanding clinician perception of common presentations in south Asians seeking mental health treatment and determining barriers and facilitators to treatment. *Asian Journal of Psychiatry, 7*, 15–21.

Razali, S. M., Khan, U. A., & Hasanah, C. I. (1996). Belief in supernatural causes of mental distress among Malay patients: Impact on treatment. *Acta Psychiatrica Scandinavica, 94*(4), 229–233. https://doi.org/10.1111/j.1600-0447.1996.tb09854.x.

Reddy, M. V., & Chandrasekhar, C. R. (1998). Prevalence of mental and behavioral disorders in India: A met analysis. *Indian Journal of Psychiatry, 40*, 149–157.

Regmi, S. K., Pokhsarel, A., Ojha, S. P., et al. (2004). Nepal mental health country profile. *International Review of Psychiatry, 16*, 142–149.

Risdal, D., & Singer, G. H. S. (2004). Marital adjustment in parents of children with disabilities: A historical review and meta-analysis. *Research & Practice for Persons with Severe Disabilities, 29*, 95–103.

Rodrigo, C., Fernando, T., Rajapakse, S., Silva, V. D., & Hanwella, R. (2013). Caregiver strain and symptoms of depression among principal caregivers of patients with schizophrenia and bipolar affective disorder in Sri Lanka. *International Journal of Mental Health Systems, 7*, 2.

Romans, S. E., & Seemans, M. V. (2013). *Women's mental health: A lifecycle approach*. Philadelphia: LWW.

Rueve, M. E., & Welton, R. S. (2008). Violence and mental distress. *Psychiatry, 5*(5), 34–48. Retrived from https://www.ncbi.nlm.nih.gov/pmc/articles/PMC2686644/

Saeed, K., Gater, R., Hussain, A., & Mubbashar, M. (2000). The prevalence, classification and treatment of mental disorders among attenders of native faith healers in rural Pakistan. *Social Psychiatry and Psychiatric Epidemiology, 35*(10), 480–485.

Sahithya, B. R., & Reddy, R. (2018). Burden of mental distress: A review in an Indian context. *International Journal of Culture and Mental Health, 11*(1), 1–11. https://doi.org/10.1080/17542863.2018.1442869.

Salib, E., & Youakim, S. (2001). Spiritual healing in elderly psychiatric patients: A case-control study in an Egyptian psychiatric hospital. *Aging & Mental Health, 5*, 366–370. https://doi.org/10.1080/13607860120080323.

Samy, A. L., Khalaf, Z. F., & Low, W. Y. (2015). Mental health in the Asia-Pacific region: An overview. *The Journal of Behavioral Science, 10*(2), 9–18.

Schuler, S. R., & Nazneen, S. (2018). Does intimate partner violence decline as Women's empowerment becomes normative? Perspectives of Bangladeshi women. *World Development, 101*, 284–292. https://doi.org/10.1016/j.worlddev.2017.09.005.

Schuler, S. R., Lenzi, R., Nazneen, S., & Bates, L. M. (2013). Perceived decline in intimate partner violence against women in Bangladesh: Qualitative evidence. *Studies in Family Planning, 44*(3), 243–257.

Sharma, B., & Slate, J. R. (2013). Recognizing the diversity in the asian population. *International Journal of Psychology Research: Hauppauge, 8*(4), 269–289.
Sharma, I., Pandit, B., Pathak, A., & Sharma, R. (2013). Hinduism, marriage and mental illness. *Indian Journal of Psychiatry, 55*(Suppl 2), S243.
Simkhada, P., Van Teijlingen, E., & Marahatta, S. B. (2015). Mental health services in Nepal: Is it too late? *Journal of Manmohan Memorial Institute of Health Sciences, 1*(4), 1–2.
Somasundaram, O., & Ratnaraj, P. (2018). Kilpauk mental hospital: The Bethlem of South Asia – A recall of its history prior to 1970. *Indian Journal of Psychiatry, 60*(2), 183–191.
Srivastava, A. (2013). Marriage as a perceived panacea to mental distress in India: Reality check. *Indian Journal of Psychiatry, 55*(Suppl 2), S239–S242.
Subba, S. H., Binu, V. S., Menezes, R. G., Kanchan, T., Arun, M., Patil, R., et al. (2009). Pattern and trend of deliberate self-harm in Western Nepal. *Journal of Forensic Sciences, 54*(3), 704–707.
Swaminath, G., & Bhide, A. (2009). 'Cinemadness': In search of sanity in films. *Indian Journal of Psychiatry, 51*(4), 244–246. https://doi.org/10.4103/0019-5545.58287.
Szymanski, D. M., & Henning, S. M. (2007). The role of self-objectification in women's depression: A test of objectification theory. *Sex Roles, 56*(1), 45–53.
Thara, R., & Padmavati, R. (2013). Community mental health care in South Asia. *World Psychiatry, 12*(2), 176.
Thara, R., & Patel, V. (1998). Women's mental health: A public health concern. *Regional Health Forum WHO South-East Asia Region, 5*, 1.
Tipping, G., & Segall, M. (1995). *Health care seeking behavior in developing countries: an annotated bibliography and literature review development bibliography*. Brighton: Institute of Development Studies, Sussex University.
Trivedi, J. K., Mishra, M., & Kendurkar, A. (2007). Depression among women in the south-Asian region: The underlying issues. *Journal of Affective Disorders, 102*(1–3), 219–225.
Trivedi, J. K., Sareen, H., & Dhyani, M. (2009). Psychological aspects of widowhood and divorce. *Mens sana monographs, 7*(1), 37.
Vijayakumar, L. (2004). *Suicide prevention meeting the challenge together*. Chennai: Orient Longman.
Walaa, M. S., & Vohra, A. (2013). Role of islam in the management of psychiatric disorders. *Indian Journal of Psychiatry, 55*(Suppl 2), S205–S214. https://doi.org/10.4103/0019-5545.105534.
Wales, J., Brewin, N., Raghavan, R., & Arcelus, J. (2017). Exploring barriers to south asian help-seeking for eating disorders. *Mental Health Review Journal, 22*(1), 40–50.
World Health Organization. (2000). *Women's mental health: An evidence based review* (No. WHO/MSD/MDP/00.1). Geneva: World Health Organization.
World Health Organization. (2015). *Investing in mental health*. Retrieved from https://www.who.int/mental_health/media/investing_mnh.pdf
Yu, S. (2018). Uncovering the hidden impacts of inequality on mental health: A global study. *Translational Psychiatry, 8*(1), 98. https://doi.org/10.1038/s41398-018-0148-0.
Zafar, M., & Malik, A. S. (2016). A study of urban women's reproductive health decisions within socio-cultural context of Pakistan. *Pakistan Journal of Women's Studies= Alam-e-Niswan= Alam-i Nisvan, 23*(2), 115.

Chapter 8
The Political Sociology of South Asian Women's Health

Farooq Hasnat, Sara Rizvi Jafree, Ainul Momina, and Zamurrad Awan

8.1 Introduction

The sociology of political systems of South Asia and its influence on women's health behaviour and health outcomes has been a neglected area in research. One of the basic premises of political sociology is the recognition that politicians and public officials are socially accountable for the provision of adequate, efficient, and equitable health services for different women's groups (Janoski et al. 2005). Where the sociology of health is important for helping us consider that social factors determine health, such as gender, class, wealth, ethnicity, and literacy, it is the sociology of politics that helps us identify that public health policy is instrumental in closing the social gaps of health inequality. In the capitalist democracies of the modern world, health is political because the planning and distribution of public health services is dependent on political intervention and also because some social groups have more access compared to others (Bambra et al. 2005). The role of the state becomes more important especially in conservative and traditional milieus like South Asia where regressive cultural forces prevent women from maintaining optimal health or seeking health recovery. Without state responsibility for health policy and social policy management for the women of South Asia, there is little possibility for diverse women groups in the region to attain holistic health quality of lives.

Pressure on the governments of the world started post the 1980s when public healthcare became a global concern, driven by capitalist forces (Porter 2005).

F. Hasnat · Z. Awan
Department of Political Science, Forman Christian College University, Lahore, Pakistan

S. R. Jafree
Department of Sociology, Forman Christian College University, Lahore, Pakistan

A. Momina (✉)
King Edward Medical University, Lahore, Pakistan

S. R. Jafree (ed.), *The Sociology of South Asian Women's Health*,
https://doi.org/10.1007/978-3-030-50204-1_8

Success and failure of governments and the nation became linked with the demands of capitalism for healthy and tireless women performing the triple shift and working both at home and in the workforce. Health specialities, health services, and medical drugs were developed for women, especially with regard to their reproductive health (Berro Pizzarossa 2018). Medical intervention for women also served as a motive for expanding capitalist profit. The governments of the region have shown commitment by participating in worldwide conferences and signing international charters to plan and implement more effective policies for safeguarding the health of their women populations.[1] Despite all this, key indicators of health for women are still not very promising in the South Asian region. As a group, South Asian countries rank second to last for gender equality (World Economic Forum 2017). Pakistan, India, Bhutan, and Sri Lanka have seen a widening of the gender gap, and of greater concern is that health and survival gaps have increased in India, Bhutan, and Pakistan.

Politicians from the developed world have won votes for promising their electorate improvements in health, including more specialized areas such as mental health, dental health, and dementia (Roberts et al. 2003). Conversely, in the democracies of South Asia, competing political parties are still lobbying for votes based on religion, ethnicity, province, caste, or class, and the function of political activity has been limited to the formation of government (Vergne 2009). Citizenship accountability for the political role in the management of community and distribution of scarce resources to all social groups has been non-existent. Powerful political parties and military rule have suppressed public expectations for public health and ignored women's health needs. Since South Asian women have always been weaker citizens of the state, they have been unable to hold their elected government officials responsible for health delivery or engage with powerful male actors to mobilize political initiatives for women's health policies. Only when politicians are elected based on their plans for the health sector and then held accountable for public health service delivery will women and other marginalized groups benefit.

The patriarchal and feudal systems of South Asia have for centuries sidelined women from policy representation and governance participation (United Nations-Economic and Social Commission for Asia and the Pacific 2007). South Asian countries suffer from post-colonial problems that have influenced women's integration and development across the structures of society, most especially the health sector (Ziltener and Künzler 2013). Significant barriers such as corruption, low-budget allocations, and deprioritized agendas have made the prioritization of women's health policies a critically neglected area. Many of the developments for

[1] This includes the Fourth World Conference on Women (Beijing, 1995), the International Conference on Population and Development (ICPD-Cairo,1994), the World Conference on Human Rights (Vienna,1993), and the World Health Organization's Health For All strategy. South Asian countries are also signatories of the Convention on the Elimination of All Forms of Discrimination Against Women (CEDAW), under which they are entitled to ensure equitable healthcare services for all women populations. Furthermore, by adopting the Millennium Development Goals, South Asian countries are now liable to achieve targets for maternal and child health and poverty alleviation of women.

women's health are a consequence of indigenous women taking over from the legacies left behind by colonial rulers, for example, in studying medicine and nursing, specializing in gynaecology, and teaching in medical schools. Since independence, with the growing chains of democratization, the return of traditional values, and the revival of extremist religious groups, developments for women's health have not shown significant progress. Furthermore, there is little consideration for marginalized women populations, like girls, ageing women, working women, and single women, who are at even greater risk for health problems due to extreme social and environmental factors. Health policies for women and other marginalized groups of society including the disabled, the third gender, and the displaced women populations are almost non-existent. Heterogeneous women's development groups across the South Asian region have not pressurized policymakers to target women's health programmes, in order to preserve religious and cultural sentiments. This may partially be because of the pressing concerns of regional conflict, natural disasters, and economic instability, but it is also because of the sidelining of women from public policy altogether.

8.2 Political Representation

South Asian women are critically under-represented in national parliament (in Bangladesh, 20.3% of women hold seats in national parliament; India, 11.8%; Pakistan, 20.6%; and Sri Lanka, 5.8%) (Asian Development Bank 2018), and less than 10% of the ministers in the region are women (United Nations 2010). As women's reserve seats for political representation are not balanced for the population, women are mostly dependent on men for mapping and mobilization of women's health policies. Generally, there is failure to create effective pressure because women citizens of South Asia are unaware that their public representatives are responsible for ensuring that they receive basic health rights along with other citizenship rights. In addition, there is also the problem of lack of awareness in majority of the illiterate and semi-literate women populations of South Asia and their ability to hold political representatives accountable for formal and informal action.[2]

The professional climate for political participation in South Asia is male-dominated, corrupt, and dependent on powerful male networks and kinship (Waylen 2005). Not only do majority women feel uncomfortable and unsafe in political office, but also they are unable to balance the home-work equation in the slow and inefficient bureaucratic structures. The lack of promotion opportunities and chances for effective governance participation for women in public offices is also a disincentive for women to invest in efforts for political vocations. Due to international pressure, gender quotas have been introduced in South Asian parliaments, and this has

[2] Formal accountability regarding health includes health budgets, access to primary healthcare, and health regulation and quality; whereas, informal accountability includes factors like commitment, ethics, and professionalism.

helped manifest representation (Rai et al. 2006), but there are serious issues to consider with regard to policy mobilization for women's rights and nepotistic and ethnic placement of women in public office as tokens.[3] Despite the steady increase in the number of South Asian women who are voting, men are still more involved in political activity and political decisions. Male voices are heard, and public policy is adopted to suit their needs. More commonly, it is believed that the supply of South Asian women in public office and political bureaucracy is low due to structural barriers imposed by the conservative culture and capitalist patriarchy. However, there is also a sociocultural role of women perception for candidacy. South Asian women do not consider themselves qualified or professionally capable for political office (Krook and Norris 2014).

Election campaigning for women in South Asia is extremely difficult, unless they have a family background in politics and are lobbying for emotional votes based on nepotism (Iwanaga 2008). The women who have campaigned and won elections in South Asia have rarely included feminist agendas or women's health objectives in their campaign. In fact, women politicians of South Asia have made a conscious effort to distance themselves from feminist attitudes in order to secure support from the more instrumental male constituency and avoid a reaction from politico-religious and other conservative groups. There is no doubt that feminist drives and women's health agendas are frowned upon by conservative male populations of South Asia, despite the change in attitudes across the world.

8.3 Government Budget for Health

There is no unanimous political system across South Asia (Baxter 2002). Interestingly, the country that ranks the best for health outcomes for women, Sri Lanka, leans towards a centralized power with presidency control. Bangladesh and Pakistan have had a complicated history with democracy being disrupted by military dictatorship. India seems to have established a secular democracy, but like Pakistan, the political culture has strong undercurrents of religious influence on political decisions and women development policies. The period before the 1970s had strong state-driven economic planning across South Asia, dominated by government ownership and intervention. However, post the 1980s, following global trends, most South Asian states started to favour privatization and deregulation of the economy, including the health sector (Haque 2003). Plagued by an illusion of democracy, majority of women do not have a political voice in South Asia (Omvedt 2005). Though women are increasingly being used to secure votes, they remain separated from policy mobilization.

[3] The theory of tokenism describes how a few women are employed and used in inferior positions to show the gender neutrality of the company, but in actuality, it is the men who retain the better positions and a larger share of remuneration.

As a result, public expenditure in key health areas for women such as social campaigning, health awareness, costs of drugs and consultancy, and subsidization for health services has remained limited (Chakraborty 2016;Maitra and Mukhopadhyay 2012). Women from poorer backgrounds, rural areas, and inferior ethnicities remain even more powerless. Impoverished women who are solely dependent on public healthcare services are suffering due to the lack of access, equity, and low-quality services. Though the citizen report cards in India and Bangladesh have been a voice for disadvantaged and rural communities, the enforcement of change and consistency in data collection is still not satisfactory (Ahmed et al. 2016). In fact, the results of recent public attitudes towards the improvement of health services in Bangladesh are unsatisfactory (Osman 2008). This is because policy mobilizers and report interpreters are men and the changes needed are cultural in nature. Additionally, small-scale and community-based interventions do not benefit the large population base.

Despite great poverty and shortfall of rural healthcare services by the private sector, the public health sector delivers services to an average of only 30% of the South Asian population (Haque 2003) (Bangladesh, 36.6% of public sector provision in healthcare services; India, 31%; and Pakistan, 27%) (Ahmed et al. 2016). This is an indicator of great deprivation for the impoverished, rural, and lower-middle-class people of the South Asian region, who comprise more than 70% of the population. The average growth rate for GDPs across South Asia is about 5.7% (Haque 2003), with government expenditure as a percentage of GDP averaging 16%. Though the government budgets are not insignificant, South Asian governments are lagging far behind developed and welfare countries in allocating state budgets for health services; for example, Sweden spends 9.2% of its GDP on health services (Bangladesh, 0.3% of government expenditure on health as a percentage of GDP; India, 1.3%; Pakistan, 2.1%; and Sri Lank, 1.5%) (Engelgau et al. 2011). As a result, the provision of access, efficiency, and accountability for the South Asian public sector is extremely inadequate. Areas such as patient record keeping, error reporting, and sufficient health resources are specifically unsatisfactory. Most of the governments are doing little to alleviate external debts, and there is great dependency on foreign aid and investment for the healthcare of women.

For South Asian citizens who can afford it, there is greater preference for private health centres due to lack of access and quality of public health centres (Basu et al. 2012). As financial protection is not available for majority populations, private healthcare can cause distress financing which contributes to growing poverty in the region. Women patients of heart disease and cancer are specifically at greater risk of indebtedness and impoverishment (Kastor and Mohanty 2018). Additionally, commodification of health in the capitalist world has made health access expensive for women whilst providing more choices and opportunities for the financially and socially empowered men (Bambra et al. 2005). Even in urban spaces, the utilization of healthcare facilities is low for women from the poorer and lower-middle-class families. Inadequate health facilities because of poor management and weak infrastructure at public hospitals further create disincentives for both the deprived classes and the privileged. This is why in most South Asian countries, private healthcare is accessed more than public healthcare.Though India and Bangladesh claim to have attained better health technologies and medical equipment, the higher cost has limited access to the rich and upper classes (Chakravarthi 2013;Islam and Biswas 2014).

The availability of healthcare resources and medical practitioners is critically inadequate in the region, with the doctor-to-population ratios much lower than the minimum international standards recommended by WHO of 1:1000 (Bangladesh, 0.47 doctor per 1000 population; India, 0.76:1000; Pakistan, 0.98:1000; and Sri Lanka, 0.88:1000) (Asian Development Bank 2018). Similarly, there are serious shortages in hospital beds for inpatient population (Bangladesh, 0.8 hospital beds per 1000 population; India, 0.7; Pakistan, 0.6; and Sri Lanka, 3.5) (Asian Development Bank 2018). Not only are enrolment and scholarships for healthcare studies low, but there is very little public sector capacity to absorb healthcare students in the region. Additionally, due to unsatisfactory work environments and inadequate compensation, there is a brain drain of the already short supply of health practitioners in South Asia. Patriarchal norms have created social barriers specifically against women health practitioners from entering into the non-segregated health workforce, including (i) women doctors who are not allowed to work in the profession after graduating and (ii) women not getting permission to study in perceived lower status health professions such as nursing, physiotherapy, and community health.

Numerous health occupations that are understaffed and thus ineffective in South Asia include health planning, health monitoring, health research, public medical and nursing schools, public hospitals and practitioners, and health social workers. South Asian countries are still struggling to deal with weak primary healthcare facilities (van Weel et al. 2016). As many primary health services can be provided by non-physicians, there is great need for the training of non-physician practitioners to fill the vacuum created by physician shortages. Non-physician practitioners include nurses and health management professionals, like public health graduates (Tiwari et al. 2018). Linking graduate programs in universities with health sector jobs is a direction that South Asian countries need to move towards. Graduates of social work, sociology, public health, and health administration need to be encouraged and then provided opportunities for employment in the health sector to provide primary healthcare and administrative support to reduce critical shortages. Expansion in the health workforce overall and specifically women practitioners would mean an increase in jobs for both men and women (Misau et al. 2010). An increase in women healthcare practitioners in South Asia would also mean an increase in quality care services and patient safety (Tong 1998).

It is widely agreed that health research is the most important driver behind health gains and patient recovery (Yazbeck and Peters 2003). If we view the health structure as a subsystem of the wider economy, familiar patterns of gender inequality will surface to help us understand why women's health research has not been a priority. The scarce health budget and domination of male health practitioners and male policymakers have sidelined health research altogether, with heavy dependence on emulating health research from the West (Swaminathan et al. 2017). As there is great poverty in South Asian countries, research-based health policymaking is even more important in the region to develop plans for not only health policy but also health financing. Support and funding of scientific research and innovation by the South Asian governments is the key factor to sustained and region-specific growth and development. However, the government budget allocations for research and innovation in the region are very low (India = 0.62% of GDP is allocated for research and development; Pakistan = 0.25%; and Sri Lanka = 0.10%) (Engelgau et al. 2011). In addition, there are few researchers in the country and even fewer gender-based health researchers to help assess and recommend health improvements for women (India, 404 researchers per million inhabitants; Pakistan, 536; and Sri Lanka, 248) (Engelgau et al. 2011).

Most of the research on women's health revolves around the body and not on the sociology of women's health or on public policies for women's health (Annandale 2005, 2008). This is especially true for South Asia, where patriarchal norms focus on using healthcare and developing health services to control reproduction and female fecundity. This is why there is negligence for health problems related to mental health, communicable and non-communicable diseases, and injury-induced health problems. Two problems that are crippling the intervention of public health policy-makers in South Asia is that first, we are dependent on health research from the West and, second, we are dependent on private bodies for medical research and technology development. The latter includes the professional dominance and occupational interests of medical practitioners and pharmaceutical companies; which necessitates the involvement of public research centres to step forward for women's health research (Latten et al. 2018;Light 2007). South Asian governments need to take immediate initiative for investment in research for the health needs of South Asian women, as their health challenges and recovery options are different compared to women from other regions of the world.

8.4 Government Licensing, Regulation, and Honesty

The depoliticization of health has occurred through the dominance of the medical model (Larson 1999). The dominant ideology is that when a woman is sick, she will visit the medical practitioner and take the relevant medical drugs to get better. In this exchange, the practitioner and the pharmaceutical company are all-powerful. Patients and public officials are made to believe that they have no control over health maintenance and recovery. In South Asian countries, most healthcare practitioners and pharmaceutical companies are able to assign disease, fix drug prices, and provide health services and drugs that are not regulated or monitored by the government as comprehensively and consistently as they should be (Brhlikova et al. 2011).

Access to and appropriate use of medicine is amongst the major health sector problems in most of the developing countries. Along with lack of investment in human resources for the health sector, the pharmaceutical profession seriously lacks government interest in Pakistan (Azhar et al. 2009). The healthcare system without pharmacists is unable to cope effectively with most medicine-related issues. Thus, involvement of skilled and authoritative pharmacists in therapeutic procedures is necessary to improve appropriate use of medicines, eliminate medication errors, make proper use of the medicine budget by efficient management (to ensure maximum access), and ensure the implementation of National Essential Medicine List (NEML). There is fear about the promotion of complementary and alternative medicine in South Asian states. The Indian government has established the ministry of "AYUSH" to promote practices like Ayurveda and yoga to help in dealing with an array of health conditions (Chopra et al. 2013). However, alternative medicine, including Ayurveda, is known to have harmful ingredients with adverse effects, and government monitoring for use in the country is a concern.

The inefficacy of the state health licensing and regulatory system can adversely influence the health outcomes of the people and influence patient mortality negatively (Blair and Durrance 2014;Morgan and Ensor 2016). As women are the more secluded and unaware gender, they are more at risk of unlicensed practitioners and unregistered drugs. State regulation is crucial to ensure the unification of interests of multiple stakeholders. Health centres, practitioner colleges and training institutes, and pharmaceutical industries are responsible for health outcomes, but they do not have unified interests. The lack of state regulation of medical centres, medical colleges, and pharmaceutical companies means that they not only operate for profit maximization but also services are compromised due to absence of accountability. Some of the main areas where South Asian public health regulatory policy falls short include patient safety standards, error reporting, patient records, quality drugs, practitioner licensing, and resource adequacy. Also, the capacity of South Asian governments to manage and reduce national health risks and be prepared for health emergencies is not satisfactory (Bangladesh, 78% of international standards for health regulations have been implemented; India, 95%; Pakistan, 51%; and Sri Lanka, 76%) (World Health Organization 2018). The figures imply that citizens have little trust in the state to support them during national emergencies. Research shows that when trust is built by improved state regulation, health behaviour improves due to increased confidence in the system (Brhlikova et al. 2011).

One of the salient cultural forces in South Asia is the rejection of the Western biomedical model and the dependency on complementary healthcare (Bodeker and Ong 2005). In fact, there is state sanction in South Asia for the use of complementary healthcare including homoeopathy, Ayurveda, and Unani. There is also little government resistance to traditional Hakeem medicine and the practice of untrained local midwives. The problem here is not the use of alternative medicine, but the lack of quality control and regulation of alternative medicine and complementary providers. Religious and traditional support for alternative medicine and traditional practitioners is so strong that it compels the state to detach itself from its responsibility. To complicate the problem, the conservative climate that operates in South Asia compels the women to opt for alternative health services, as they are: (i) available within the neighbourhood and do not require women to travel far or undergo physical examinations, (ii) usually non-invasive health solutions, (iii) perceived as more trustworthy due to traditional use by previous generations, and (iv) cheaper than biomedicine.

The governments of South Asia have always considered the management of women's health affairs to be a private domain, to be decided and executed by family traditions, tribal customs, and religious interpretations. In all, acquiescence to complementary healthcare in South Asia has loosened state liability for not only women's health outcomes and women's health policy but also regulation and quality control for the health structure. Alternative medicine has its risks of reducing choices for treatment and opting for irrational recovery options leading to mortality (Angell and Kassirer 1998). Regulation of complementary medicine is critical to prevent adverse consequences for women's health and maternal health, ranging from damage to the immune system and other body organs, bleeding and hypoglycaemia, hormonal and gynaecological side effects from oral contraception, extreme sedation and hypertension, and aggravation of mental illness (Kramlich 2014).

South Asian countries are also greatly influenced by drug abuse, with women almost matching the statistics for male drug use (Kensy et al. 2012). Without government intervention for illicit drug use, there is risk of drug overuse, drug dependency, and higher mortality. It must be recognized that women who are unable to access healthcare services, or face discrimination from the health sector, may turn to drug abuse to seek pain relief or other health solutions. Marginalized women populations who consume illicit drugs include those who: (i) suffer greater economic deprivation, (ii) do not receive symmetrical assistance for domestic burdens, (iii) have mental health problems, (iv) work in the sex trade, and (v) are ethnic minorities.

Social customs of South Asia suggest that when there is group drug abuse, women are injected last and, as poorer members of the community, they are at risk of consuming low-quality cheaper drugs, leading to even greater risk of diseases (Kensy et al. 2012). The consequences of drug abuse in women take on a more sinister shape when we consider that women are the primary nurturers of children and stabilizers of the family. Pregnant women of South Asia have been found to consume opium for its sedation benefits, with risks to preterm delivery and compromised foetus (Maghsoudlou et al. 2018;Ray et al. 2006). There needs to be strict government accountability and legal protection for children in South Asia by monitoring and penalizing drug abuse during pregnancy. The impact that drug abuse has on a mother's physical and emotional health and the development of children must be considered by the state as part of child protection policies. Women who consume drugs in South Asia face greater stigmatization, due to the patriarchal beliefs that women are the emotional buttress and primary nurturers for the family and children. Generally, greater drug abuse in the family and community, even when the women are non-consumers, means greater risk of sexually transmitted diseases, violence, and abuse against women.

Opiates and amphetamine-type stimulants are the two major sources of drug abuse in the region. Pakistan and India are known to produce illicit opium with great consequences to the health of their populations such as drug dependency and adverse health consequences (Drugs and Crime 2010). What the government must also consider is that opium cultivation has become an important financial source for a significant number of South Asian women. More women in South Asia are getting involved in drug trafficking due to coercion by male family members, as there is less suspicion attached to women in criminal activities. The state also needs to consider that incarceration of women drug traffickers has consequences for children, who might have to serve jail sentence with their mothers or be left at home alone without a mother's care. South Asian governments need to plan better laws for different levels of involvement, reasons for involvement, and imprisonment for women with children.

On the surface, it seems that the problem with inefficient public health services is the lack of funds and government budget. However, there is a case of South Asia having some of the richest politicians in the world and having high rates of corruption in politics and bureaucracy (Haque 2003). Rich politicians in poor countries of South Asia may be deprioritizing health policy as they do not want to rechannel finances for the maintenance of elite political bureaucracy and capitalistic agendas. Improved transparency, accountability, and audit of the politicians and the public healthcare systems in South Asia are imperative for demarginalization of women's health policy. Corrupt practices in the health sectors of the region that are common and embedded in the substructures, include: (i) embezzlement and bribery, (ii) lack of error reporting and adherence to patient safety practices, (iii) medical quackery and regulation of practitioner and drugs, and (iv) poor service delivery and monitoring of medical practice. The system of corruption starts from the medical colleges, with bribes being given for admission of non-merit-based students and also for passing of medical examinations. This unmeritocratic selection and licensing of medical practitioners contribute to poor service delivery and low patient safety standards across South Asia.

Public sector patients suffer not only due to the low competency of the practitioner but also due to the corruption of practitioners in: (i) spending more time in private practice for profit earning and not fulfilling government job hours, (ii) using public medical equipment for private practices, and (iii) streaming patients into the private sector to make money (Lewis 2006;Punjani et al. 2014). The distribution and circulation of out of stock and banned or low-quality drugs is a common occurrence, and it usually occurs because of the corruption of state quality control officers. The trading of human organs is also rampant in South Asia, as deprived and impoverished populations are exploited for large amounts of money involved in organ trafficking (Scheper-Hughes et al. 2000). Most specifically women have suffered due to the corruption in the health sector. The unregulated commercialization of medical intervention has meant many women are forced into C-sections, invasive procedures, and expensive tests that they might not need (Carroll 2017). Additionally, lack of surveillance and monitoring has meant that many women, as the subordinate gender, suffer from violence, abuse, and neglect from healthcare practitioners (Niaz 2003). Women are more vulnerable targets as they are less likely to respond to or report neglect and abuse. Different forms of violence such as rape, physical assault, and harassment are common not only against women patients but also women healthcare providers of South Asia, including women doctors, nurses, paramedical staff, physiotherapists, and lady healthcare workers (Jafree 2018). Consequently, women are unwilling to seek services or work in the health sector, be it the clinical zones, teaching centres, or in community spaces. Ultimately, awareness of corruption in the health sector has influenced the choice of women patients, in that many do not seek health services due to belief in fraudulent treatment, inferior care, and questionable treatment options.

Licensed and legitimate practitioners and administrators of the health sector are also suffering due to state corruption (Economakis et al. 2010). Corruption in the health budget and low fund allocations means that practitioners are: (i) underpaid and undertrained, (ii) having to work in unsatisfactory organizational culture with poor resources, and (iii) not getting equal compensation for their services. This leads to low incentives for practitioners to perform their roles optimally and has also contributed to a large brain drain and immigration of healthcare practitioners from South Asia. Law enforcement and policies against corruption are inadequate in the region, and most elite groups are able to manipulate the government and constitution to favour their interests at the cost of the health needs of the majority population. When governments make efforts to eradicate corruption in the health sector, practitioner performance, patient safety, and national health improve collectively.

8.5 Skewed Population Ratios

The population of South Asia has crossed over 1 and a half billion people, and despite the large human resource strength, the governments have been unable to encash the demographic dividend (Dasvarma 2003). The emphasis has been on recognizing the structural discrepancies across different populations in the rural spaces, feudal areas, tribal zones, and desert and mountainous zones. No doubt, the large population base requires critical planning and systematic assessment for the management of the health programs, specifically for the subordinate genders. However, less attention has been given to the burden of patriarchy within the households and communities which has contributed to the "missing women" in South Asia (Gupta 2005). With approximately 106 men to a 100 women living in the region (United Nations 2010), the sex ratio for South Asia is more skewed towards the men compared to any other region of the world. The social reason for this masculinization of sex ratios includes the traditional and rigid preference for sons. Millions of women are prevented from being born in the region, through female foeticide, and countless are wiped out during the first 5 years of their life. The less than 5 years child mortality for the daughters of South Asia is greater than that of sons (Bangladesh, 30.0 female deaths per 1000 live births; India, 40.4; Pakistan = 71.2; and Sri Lanka, 08.0) (World Bank Group 2014).

Discriminatory and male-dominated politico-legal structures have neglected to consider public policies to prevent female foeticide or reduce girl child mortality. South Asian women forced to abort the female foetus after gender-determining ultrasounds are less able to seek legal recourses or adopt political networking to save their child's life. Many women, burdened and conditioned by patriarchy, choose to abort their female foetus in order to prevent violence against themselves and save any future daughters from abuse and neglect. Female foeticide and mortality rates for girls in the region highlight an unnatural characteristic of South Asian mothers. It is not normal or familiar for mothers to kill their child (Friedman and Resnick 2007), but mothers in South Asia are habituated to believe that daughters will become a vessel for their dishonour and shame. There is little recognition for mothers in the region who make choices or are forced for foetal abortions and the consequent emotional and psychological problems they suffer from.

State policy and awareness campaigns have still not effectively infiltrated cultural patterns of allocating higher social status to sons. As a result, boys comparatively receive better nutrition and care from the family during the critical first 5 years of life (Hazarika 2000;Mishra et al. 2004). They also receive more immediate medical attention and hospital check-ups with trained practitioners in the event of an illness, as the money and time spent on a son's health are considered a worthy investment for the future. The consequences of imbalanced gender ratios in South Asia are immense and sinister and unaccounted for by the government; they include: (i) the sustenance of patriarchy, (ii) fewer women to marry and reproduce and thus a greater burden on existing women to produce multiple children, and (iii) an increase in crime, drug use, and deviant sexual behaviour due to an increase in younger men (Dyson 2012).

The rural women face greater problems due to sex-selective abortions and girl child mortality (Sudha and Rajan 1999). This is because regressive cultural forces against women are stronger in the rural areas, resulting in greater health deprivation for abortion care, birth spacing, and mental health. South Asia has a large rural-based population which faces problems related to access and quality of healthcare services (Bangladesh, 64.1% of the population are rural based; India, 66.4%; Pakistan, 63.6%; and Sri Lanka, 80.6%) (Asian Development Bank 2018). As the private sector does not find rural spaces to be commercially attractive for profit maintenance, there is shortfall and low quality of primary healthcare services by the public sector in the rural areas of South Asia (Zaidi et al. 2017). In the absence of tertiary and secondary public healthcare services, most rural populations have to travel great distances for their health needs leading to higher mortality and delayed detection of disease. This is why rural maternal mortality ratios are worst compared to the urban ratios, with little evidence of other health indicator comparisons for women between the two zones (Bhutta et al. 2004).

8.6 Poverty and Health Financing

Approximately 40% of the world's poor reside in the region, with more women compared to men comprising the impoverished. Ranked as the lower-income countries of the world, by the World Bank, the women of South Asia have an average income per day estimated at USD 2.7–10.8 (World Economic Forum 2017). Women of the region are unable to emerge from the cycle of poverty primarily because of disadvantages in inheritance and property rights and also informal sector employment (United Nations 2010). Absence of house ownership, land entitlements, and savings bonds render women not only with lower status in the family, but also there is less investment by the family for their health needs.

Only 36% of South Asian women are part of the labour force (United Nations 2010). Unemployment for women is still high due to cultural beliefs that women are to be secluded and reserved for reproduction and home care (Bangladesh, 6.7% of women above the age of 15 years are unemployed; India, 3.7%; and Pakistan = 6.1%) (Asian Development Bank 2018). Of concern is that full and productive employment for women is the first step for their autonomous decision-making related to health. Majority of unemployed women in South Asia do not have social protection from the government with regard to unemployment benefits and health coverage (Kuhn et al. 2018). Unemployed women in the region have been presumed to be covered in health through public health schemes, reproductive health policies, and employment policies of husbands or fathers. However, this has relegated women as dependents for health access and care and deprived them of comprehensive health services. The state now needs to stop planning for women as dependents and instead recognize them as individuals with basic health needs and rights.

The proportion of employed women in South Asia living below the international line of poverty is far greater than other parts of the world (Bangladesh, 46.6% of women live below the line of poverty; India, 12.3%; Pakistan, 4.7%; and Sri Lanka, 1%) (Asian Development Bank 2018). Very few women in South Asia are represented in the top managerial positions, confirming that they do not have much influence over organizational and corporate sector decision-making or managerial policies for women's equality (Bangladesh, 11.5% of women in managerial positions; India, 12.9%; Pakistan, 2.9%; and Sri Lanka, 24.8%) (Asian Development Bank 2018). Research also shows that despite employment, women of South Asia are unable to make autonomous decisions with regard to spending their income and in fact are known to hand over their earnings to the male members of their households (United Nations 2010).

Another major impediment to health access and finance for working women in South Asia is that the minority that are employed, at 80%, are working in the informal sector of the economy. Women have been used indirectly in South Asia and in other low-income nations, for foreign investment and export promotion by keeping them locked in the informal sector and low-wage occupations (Nash and Fernández-Kelly 1983;Sassen-Koob 1983). The informal sector does not provide women with employment benefits, health insurance, pension and provident funds, paid leave, or maternity benefits (Kumari and Singh 2016). Unskilled work participation for women is usually rationalized in South Asian society due to lower education and specialization of women. However, there are strong patriarchal forces preventing even highly educated and specialized women from competing with men in the formal sector such as early marriage, unsafe work environment, accepting lower pay, and reluctance to compete for higher positions for fear of competing with all-male colleagues. Across the region, nearly 22%–59% of women are married between the ages of 20–24 years, indicating that higher education, specialization, and financial autonomy are not a priority for women or that women are forced to consider marriage as their primary goal in life.

The ratio of female to male school enrolment for children aged 11–14 years in South Asian is lower than the non-South Asian states (South Asia0.70 and non-South Asian states 0.91) (Filmer and King 1999). The figures confirm that fewer girls in the region are enrolled in schools compared to boys, between the age groups of 11–14 years. This is a relevant age group to measure gender differences, as regressive cultural forces remove young girls from the education sector for reasons such as: (i) poverty, work participation, and assistance in domestic work or younger sibling care, (ii) lack of safety in the region for young girls compared to boys, (iii) association of family honour with keeping daughters closeted in the home after they cross puberty, and (iv) lack of complete segregation in girls' schools.

Women in the region form a considerable share of youth that are deprived of education, training, and employment. Literacy rates for South Asian women are well below international standards (Bangladesh 69.9% of women 15 years or older are literate; India 59.3%; Pakistan 44.3%; and Sri Lanka 90.0%) (Asian Development Bank 2018), confirming the belief that families do not prioritize retention in school for their daughters. Future employment and capability expansion are imperative for the health quality of life of women in South Asia, and the government needs to plan prudent policies for education, training, and employment of women. Of further worry is that women who are occupied in formal or informal work outside the home have little social support in receiving symmetrical household assistance (Annandale 2008). South Asian working women in both paid and unpaid employment have to pay the price of labour participation through greater burdens of disease and illness (Kane et al. 1999). As a result, they may adopt health behaviours that in the past were embraced by men to reduce work stress, including alcohol consumption, drug abuse, cigarette smoking, and the use of other harmful intoxicants. It is common to hear of women in the region suffering from coronary disease and cancer, but the emphasis on health programmes and awareness for intoxicants is usually on men and not women.

So far, South Asian state loans and income support programmes have kept women in contractual work, mostly home-based, through minimal loans with large-interest-rate loan returns (Hunt and Kasynathan 2001;Wellalage and Locke 2017). These programmes are not known to provide support for health awareness or health insurance for poor women. Instead of protecting women's health, it is not uncommon for many women to be fired or demoted if they get pregnant or get sick. More commonly found in subsidiary occupations of secretarial work or care work, women have been used to raise national production but been employed in the informal sector of the economy, which has left them bereft of health benefits and financial protection.The problem with pink-collar work and feminized professions is not only the legislative problems of less health coverage but also greater health risks due to violence and professional bullying, leading to both physical and mental health problems (Bezbaruah 2012). Additionally, women's rights groups from the region have reinforced the caring, nurturing, and community service roles in women and have not given priority to the mobilization of financial access for women with an entrepreneurial vision. Another important eco-social concern is that by cutting back on public health expenditure overall, especially for the poor, disabled, and elderly women, South Asian nations have placed an immense burden on women for unpaid care work within the homes.

Women's labour laws of South Asia need radical reform. At the moment, they do not include rights for women with regard to health, labour participation, and social security (Begum 2016). Massive efforts are needed to facilitate working mothers with regard to: (i) pay gaps between men and women, (ii) increase in maternity leave and flexible work hours, (iii) introduction of paternity relief, (as this would help cultural support for mothers), (iv) day-care centres and lactation rooms, (v) protection against dismissal or barriers to promotion for women who get married or are pregnant, and (vi) other child benefits for mothers, such as health insurance for the child and education benefits for the child. Breastfeeding is a traditionally accepted practice in South Asian society, especially amongst the poorer sections of society as breastfeeding is more affordable (Beasley and Amir 2007). However, state support for the nutritional needs of breastfeeding mothers is still a neglected area, and there is almost no employer support for organizational space and time for lactation.

The estimates for universal health coverage in South Asia are low with less than half of the people in Bangladesh and Pakistan having coverage (Bangladesh, 46% of people have health coverage; India, 56%; Pakistan, 40%; and Sri Lanka, 62%) (World Health Organization 2018). As gender constructions are rigid in the region, the traditional belief is that women are homemakers, and if they do participate in the informal sector of the economy, they do it to supplement the household income with the permission of the male members of the family. In both cases, the state neglects to recognize and define health policy for women as domestic workers and women as informal workers of the economy. Moreover, there is minimal health insurance for male workers in South Asia or their dependents, making women in the homes more vulnerable to health deprivation.

Majority of the populations of South Asia use out-of-pocket payments for health financing due to lack of health insurance provision (Yazbeck and Peters 2003). The proportion of people in South Asia with spending above 10% of total household income on health expenses is very high (Bangladesh, 13.6% of people spend more than 10% of their household income on health; India, 17.3%; Pakistan, 1.0%; and Sri Lanka, 2.9%) (World Health Organization 2018). The biggest challenge is that high dependency on health services from the private sector has translated to overproduction by the private sector and commercialization of health services. It is becoming more common for the private sector to exploit women's reproductive and gynaecological conditions and encourage costly and unnecessary interventions such as C-section, hysterectomy, hormone therapy, and invasive tests (Yazbeck and Peters 2003). There is a critical need to develop state schemes for health financing and protection of vulnerable and impoverished populations like non-working women, women working in the informal sector of the economy, the girl child, and ageing women.

Crippled by intersectional inequalities of not only gender but also race, ethnicity, class, and religion, women in South Asia are highly dependent on the state for social protection to raise their standards of living and health quality of life. At a macro level, unless women are supported in social policy for basic human needs of education, employment, and security, any isolated health sector improvements will not be effective. Women in the region are facing challenges of insecurity, demographic shortfall, and feminization of poverty, without any safety net being provided by the state. There is urgent need for social policy support from the government for unprivileged women with regard to: (i) financial support for poor women; (ii) schooling and education of women (specifically to improve retention and high education enrolment); (iii) income maintenance, skill development, and unemployment support; (iv) child protection for single mothers and families with only daughters; and (v) health access and quality of care for women of different groups (including the girl child, married women and mothers, ageing women, rural migrant women, and displaced and refugee women).

8.7 Communicable and Non-communicable Diseases and Injuries

Critically vulnerable to the triple-shift disease burden of communicable diseases, non-communicable diseases, and injuries, the death rate of South Asian women is significantly high (Bangladesh, 388 women die per 100,000 people; India, 283; Pakistan, 388; and Sri Lanka, 241) (Low et al. 2015). Specific mortality percentages for each health burden includes: (i) 46% of women from communicable diseases (including maternal and child health issues and nutrition), (ii) 41% due to non-communicable diseases, and (iii) 13% due to injuries (Engelgau et al. 2011). It is important to consider here that statistics for South Asian women's diseases have a tendency to be underreported due to lack of patient record keeping, black voids in data collection from rural and semi-literate populations, and cultural barriers to reporting health problems of women (Swaminathan et al. 2017).

The lack of commitment by South Asian governments is evident in that there is a lacklustre investment in the prevention of communicable diseases, which would result in fewer burdens on the health sector overall and less accountability on the public sector.As the subordinate gender, women are at greater risk for communicable diseases in South Asia due to greater exposure and deprivation with regard to unsafe drinking water, air pollution, and unsafe household emissions. Less than 60% of the populations of South Asia have access to safe drinking water, meaning that they are at risk of contracting multiple, but preventable diseases like-diarrhoea, typhoid, cholera, dysentery, and hepatitis (World Health Organization 2018). In about 30% of rural parts of South Asia, women are responsible for collecting water for the household (United Nations 2010), demanding a significant amount of time and resulting in less time and energy for fulfilment of other basic requirements and health needs. To multiply the burden, the water scarcity problems of South Asia are placing women in increasingly disadvantaged positions for water collection and storage (Price et al. 2014). The development of an efficient water infrastructure and safe drinking water is critically needed.

A significant number of people in South Asia suffer mortality due to high rates of air pollution (in Bangladesh,149 people per 100,000 population face mortality due to air pollution; India, 184.3; Pakistan, 173.6; and Sri Lanka 79.8) (World Health Organization 2018).Common diseases caused by air pollution include asthma, lung cancer, chronic obstructive pulmonary disease, leukaemia, pneumonia, birth defects, immune system defects, weakening lung function, and premature deaths. Women and girls are specifically at risk due to lack of social mobility (men with asthma can more easily travel to another location), higher exposure to emissions within the house, and inability to seek medical assistance due to negligence (Krishna et al. 2017). Social factors that must be managed by the state to reduce air pollution include: (i) controlling population growth, (ii) reducing and regulating industrial activity, (iii) reducing and regulating land transport and sea transport, (iv) improving policies for environmental protection, (v) planned industrialization and urbanization, and (vi) regulation for fuel burning.

Most families across South Asia use inefficient cooking stoves, polluting heating systems, and kerosene lighting for preparing meals and heating within the house. Access to clean household energy for South Asian families is critically low (in Bangladesh, 18% of people use clean fuels; India, 41%; Pakistan, 43%; and Sri Lanka, 26%) (World Health Organization 2018). Again, the burden is on the women and girls who spend long hours collecting fuel and cooking with inefficient and unhealthy supplies. As a consequence of household emissions, women are more vulnerable to health problems such as burns, poisoning, and respiratory problems (Golshan et al. 2013).

Though less researched, non-communicable diseases, including cardiovascular disease, cancer, obesity, hypertension, and diabetes are common and growing in South Asian women. Some research suggests that mortality rates for non-communicable diseases will become the leading cause of death for women in South Asia (Ghaffar et al. 2004). The DALY[4] statistics highlight the disability risks South Asian women face in the region due to non-communicable diseases (statistics for women's non-communicable diseases in South Asia: high blood glucose, 11.2% of risk; iron deficiency, 9.4%; high blood pressure, 9.1%; high cholesterol, 8.5%; and physical inactivity, 7.3%) (Engelgau et al. 2011). There are significant sociocultural factors specific to the region which place women at risk for non-communicable diseases, such as: (i) unhealthy traditional diets, (ii) undernutrition and exclusion of vegetables and fruits from diet, (iii) sedentary lifestyles and restriction to the house, (iv) limited opportunities for participation in sports and outdoor physical activity, (v) lack of financial autonomy for medication and treatment associated with chronic

[4] DALY stands for the disability-adjusted life year and represents the number of years lost due to illhealth, disease, or disability.

non-communicable diseases, (vi) overuse of tobacco and illicit drugs, and (vii) having to encounter non-communicable diseases caused by the ageing process, without savings, health protection, and state support for old-age care.

The people of South Asia are mostly found to consume traditional foods which contain oil-based gravy and other fried food, salt, white rice, refined flours, and starchy carbohydrates (Misra et al. 2008). The power of traditional eating customs is so great that even immigrant South Asian women who have been made more aware of healthier food options with access to nutritious ingredients prefer to cook and eat unhealthy meals as a form of allegiance to their culture (Garnweidner et al. 2012). There is also the problem of considerable undernourishment across the populations of South Asia, indicating complex problems of lack of awareness about healthy food and lack of money to consume nutritious foods (in Bangladesh, 15.1% of the population is undernourished; India, 14.5%; Pakistan, 19.9%; and Sri Lanka, 22.1%) (Asian Development Bank 2018).

Due to the cultural preference for sons, it is the girls and women in the households that suffer from greater rates of undernourishment in South Asia (Osmani and Sen 2003).With regard to nutritional access, research shows that the use of milk and fruit amongst women is far less than in men (Maestre and Poole 2018). Women in the region are less able to consume food items such as egg, fish, meat, and chicken, which are reserved for the men, resulting in high incidence of anaemia and undernutrition in women. Though some programmes to provide women with iron supplements during pregnancy exist (Akhtar et al. 2013), major state intervention is needed consistently across the region for the awareness and subsidization of poor families for a balanced nutritious diet.

Research shows that women who are able to participate in sports face less problems related to health and disease, including fatal and chronic illnesses such as cancer and cardiovascular disease (Reid et al. 2005). However, most women from the region choose to remain within the folds of conservatism by not participating in sports to retain the socially constructed feminine identities of submissiveness, passivity, and domestication (Benn et al. 2010). Public recreational facilities specifically for women in South Asia such as state clubs, state parks, and state sports fields are sparsely found (Nanayakkara 2012). Most state-sponsored recreation, the few that are found, caters to men and boys. Even when the intent is to fund and maintain gender-neutral recreational spaces, such as cricket grounds, football grounds, communal swimming pools, and jogging parks, these spaces eventually evolve into male-only zones. The Indian government has taken initiative to promote "AYUSH"[5]as a low-cost tool for effective prevention of disease and health therapy, but this is limited in its impact (Shrivastava et al. 2015). There needs to be compulsory inclusion of physical exercise for women in schools and the availability of exercise spaces in offices and in public spaces to promote good health for women across the region.

---

[5]AYUSH stands for the Ministry of Ayurveda, Yoga and Naturopathy, Unani, Siddha, and Homoeopathy. It is a governmental body aimed to prevent health problems through the practice of yoga and other natural therapies.

The significant tobacco consumption by women in South Asia is surprising, given that in a conservative region, women are reluctant to be associated with what is seen as a masculinized consumption pattern. What has provided opportunities for women in the region is the commonly available smokeless tobacco which can be inconspicuously chewed or snuffed (in Bangladesh, 4.0% of women tobacco users above the age of 15 years; India, 4.0%; Pakistan, 7.0%; and Sri Lanka, 2.0%) (Engelgau et al. 2011). Consequential social deprivation in women is compelling them to consume tobacco, such as: (i) dependency on intoxicants to survive difficult life circumstances (abuse, neglect, and poverty) and (ii) the lack of awareness of the health consequences of tobacco consumption. Ultimately, tobacco consumption in women has greater social consequences including serious health consequences to foetal development and the emulation of maternal practices by the children (Cnattingius 2004). Tobacco regulation and communication for awareness of health risks must be a priority for governments of South Asia.

Most neglected are the ageing women of South Asia, who commonly suffer from the dual handicap of old age diseases and poverty (Sheykhi 2007). There is absence of social security by the state for most ageing women, and they are commonly found to suffer from challenging problems like hypertension, diabetes, heart disease, musculoskeletal diseases and joint pains, renal impairment, chronic bronchitis, palpitation, dementia, and chest pain. Elderly women who are widows, separated, or divorced are especially vulnerable populations as they are bereft of guardians and care providers. Social support for ageing women is low in patriarchal setups like South Asia, mainly because elderly women are devoid of inheritance or earnings and thus do not have significant wealth or savings to pass on to their children. State subsidies do not exist for the elderly living at homes, and this provides less motivation for young adults to support their elderly for health and nutritional needs. At the same time, care must be taken to monitor the utilization of subsidies for the elderly, as some research shows that subsidies of the elderly can be taken away and misused by family members, and women of South Asia would be extremely vulnerable to this kind of abuse (Lafferty et al. 2012).

Elderly men comparatively receive more nurture and care from their families, as they control material legacies (Organization 2007). They also have their own money and resources to seek better healthcare or hire care providers when family members are unavailable or unwilling to support them during illness (Qureshi 2017). Theories of patriarchal capitalism explain how ageing men are perceived as think tanks for the economy, and thus, health investment for men is considered beneficial for the capitalist economy (Kandiyoti 1988). Prolonging men's lives and keeping them employed, in part-time consultancy roles, can reap benefits for the capitalist economy and other men. The effect of feudalism and patriarchal capitalism in South Asia may lead to decreasing gaps in life expectancy between men and women in the region, in which case the development of health policies for women, and especially ageing women, is at risk of being further sidelined in favour of health policies for men.

Overall, the medicalization of deviance has tended to liberate men but penalize women with regard to health problems, especially non-communicable diseases

(Haatanen 2015). Medical conditions and treatment for anger, depression, obesity, or sexual preferences have been more acceptable for men, compared to women. Consequently, social support and care received by men has also been greater. Where health problems such as obesity, depression, and anger have attained disease categorization, more women-health issues such as menstrual cramps and post-pregnancy depression have received no recognition or legitimacy in South Asia. As a result, women in the home and at the workplace have been deprived of assistance for home management or work leave.

Injuries of South Asian women are most commonly caused by violence, including the commonly researched physical and sexual violence, but also verbal bullying and professional bullying (Organization 2014). Bullying is known to cause mental health problems, leading to self-injury and stress-induced injuries. The non-symmetrical household burden is also a common cause of high injuries in girls and women within the household, including injuries from gas, hot water, fire stoves, lifting heavy items, and agricultural work (Golshan et al. 2013;Kelkar 2007). It must also be considered that accidental injuries in girls and women occur due to neglect, isolation, and unsafe duties required from women within the home and at the workforce in unskilled employment. Additionally, muscle injuries are caused by inadequate nutrition and diet in women (Müller and Krawinkel 2005). Regressive traditional customs exacerbate the rate of injuries and violence experienced by South Asian women, including child marriage, forced marriage, exchange marriage, kidnapping, revenge rape, attempted honour killing, dowry violence, social circumstances forcing attempted suicide, and acid burns (Niaz 2003). Though gender-based violence is a universal phenomenon, South Asian women face considerably more violence than any other region of the world due to lack of policies or policy execution (United Nations 2010).

Laws and policies to control domestic violence, workplace violence, girl-child violence, and corporal punishment are not given priority in order to appease conservatives and religious extremists in the region (Goonesekere 2004). Social conditioning includes that women should accept neglect, abuse, harassment, and violence, without seeking legal recourse or perpetrator accountability. There is no better example than culture and traditions dictating laws and policies than with the case of violence against women in South Asia. Reporting and seeking assistance is low due to unsatisfactory judicial accountability and lack of state provision for the shelter of women victims. In some regions where shelters exist, they usually do not accommodate the children of the victims, providing low incentives for mothers to escape from their disadvantaged circumstances (Niaz 2003). Disabled women experience more social exclusion and deprivation in South Asian society (Thomas and Thomas 2002). As disabled men receive preference for employment, disabled women need state support through gender-based disability quotas in private and public organizations and for political representation.

8.8 Life Expectancy and Maternal Mortality

The average gap in life expectancy for South Asian women and men is not as great as the difference in the other regions of the world (Bangladesh, 74.3% vs. 70.9% estimated life expectancy for women versus men; India, 70.2% vs. 67.1%; Pakistan, 67.5% vs. 65.5%; and Sri Lanka, 78.6% vs. 71.9%) (Engelgau et al. 2011). More importantly, the comparatively higher life expectancy figures for South Asian women lose their significance when we consider the case of the "missing women" from the region and also the fact that women spend more years with illness compared to men (Klasen and Wink 2003). Some scholars even argue that the edge that South Asian women had in life expectancy, compared to men, is slowly fading away (Annandale 2005). This is mainly because of better health services and care for men, over women.

The ratio of female to male child mortality in the region is far greater than the non-South Asian states (South Asia 1.33 and non-South Asian states 1.01) (Filmer and King 1999). The ratio shows that the girl child is more likely to die before the age of 5 years compared to the male child due to historic gender-based discrimination and negligence. This is evident in results for female-to-male children who receive no treatment for fever or acute respiratory infection in South Asian (South Asia 1.19 and non-South Asian states 1.02) (Filmer and King 1999). The ratios indicate that the daughter is less likely to receive health treatment and care when they are sick compared to sons. This extreme sociocultural discrimination against the South Asian girl child explains why girls in the region also face undernutrition and stunting (in Bangladesh, 36.1% of the children have stunted growth; India, 38.4%; Pakistan, 41.5%; and Sri Lanka, 17.3%) (Asian Development Bank 2018). Consequences of stunted growth include genetic transfer to future generations, impaired brain development, lower IQ, weakened immune system, and the consequent susceptibility to multiple diseases across the life period. Not only is state policy in South Asia non-existent to measure the comparative stunting of the girl child compared to the boy child, but there are few policies in place to support mothers with daughters.

South Asian health programmes that enforce reproductive control over the body have been rejected by men. Women, however, remain less responsive to control over their bodies due to years of ideological and authoritarian conditioning within the homes. This may be why women from the region still have some of the highest maternal mortality ratios in the world, excluding Sri Lanka (Bangladesh, 176 deaths per 100,000 live births; India, 174 deaths; Pakistan, 178 deaths; and Sri Lanka, 30 deaths) (Asian Development Bank 2018). The reasons for high maternal mortality ratios have to do with state negligence in judicious maternal and child health policies, such as: (i) raising national awareness for safe deliveries and subsidization for expectant mothers, (ii) ensuring skilled practitioners for delivery and promotion of institutional delivery, (iii) availability and utilization of prenatal and postnatal care, and (iv) supporting the transformation of cultural norms for reproductive burdens on women. In South Asia, prenatal care is still around 68%, signifying that many women and their families believe that no healthcare is needed for the planning of a safe delivery for mother and child with regard to supplementation, nutrition, and foetal monitoring (United Nations 2010). The inherent belief is that reproduction is a natural process that can take place at home and that any pregnancy complication is due to the sins of the mother (Yaya et al. 2017).

There is considerable social stigma against women who attempt to seek the services of skilled practitioners and treat their pregnancies as an "unnatural" process (El-Saharty et al. 2016). Traditional beliefs, religious fallacies, and lack of permission from husband and in-laws create barriers for access to trained practitioners. Shortage of skilled women practitioners is also a barrier as conservative families do not allow their women to seek services from male practitioners. The evidence for this lies in the underutilization of skilled practitioner services (in Bangladesh, 31.7% of women use the services of skilled practitioners for child delivery; India, 48.9%; and Pakistan, 42.1%) (Ahmed et al. 2016). Many South Asian women are still dependent on unskilled providers due to lack of access and reach (Md Illias Kanchan et al. 2017). Where community healthcare workers are functioning for the maternal health of South Asia, their efficacy is lacklustre because services are not delivered in continuity across the community due to rejection by conservative families (Bhatia 2014;Pallas et al. 2013). When lady healthcare workers (LHWs) or women community health workers face resistance in convincing male relatives and in-laws for health choices related to maternal immunization and institutional deliveries, they back away rather than stand ground to prevent violence and backlash. Low trust for biomedical health services in South Asian regions and the lack of regulation in health services have resulted in suboptimal development for the health quality of life for women.

To compound the problem, very few women opt for institutional deliveries during childbirth in South Asia (in Bangladesh, 26.9% of women opt for institutional delivery during childbirth; India, 40.4%; and Pakistan, 37.4%) (Ahmed et al. 2016). There is great fear concerning institutional deliveries and being exposed to unnecessary biomedical interventions and compromising of the traditional path expected for the mother and child (Das et al. 2016). It is feared that institutional deliveries will impose "Western" practices of immunization, birth spacing, family planning, and sterilization. Husbands and mothers-in-law of South Asia commonly attempt to prevent institutional deliveries, as it is perceived as a sinister and external force, which will empower women to take their fertility and fecundity in their own hands. Statistics for women satisfied with the use of modern methods for family planning are not as high compared to the developed regions of the world and are less than 50% for Pakistan (in Bangladesh, 72.5% of women are satisfied with their use of family planning; India, 72.0%; Pakistan, 47.0%; and Sri Lanka, 74.1%) (Asian Development Bank 2018). The figures indicate that women are unable to adequately plan their gestational period or maintain healthy gaps between pregnancies and that reproductive health policies are not prudent in protecting the women of South Asia.

A considerable number of women in South Asia are still getting married before the age of 15 years, despite international censure and awareness of the health risks (in Bangladesh, 22.4% women married before the age of 15 years; India, 6.6%; and

Pakistan, 2.8%) (Asian Development Bank 2018). The number of women married before the age of 18 years is also high (in Bangladesh, 58.6% women married before the age of 18 years; India, 27.3%; and Pakistan, 21%) (Asian Development Bank 2018). Many girls aged between 15–19 years are also giving birth in South Asia (Bangladesh, 78.0 women, between the ages of 15–19 years, per 1000 are giving birth; India, 28.1; and Pakistan, 44.0) (Asian Development Bank 2018). Though South Asian countries have developed laws to limit child marriage, the main challenge is that these laws are not implemented or enforced and the minimum age for marriage is still not above 18 years of age (Raj et al. 2012). International health guidelines state that women below the ages of 18 may still be growing and are not mentally mature for marriage (Marphatia et al. 2017). Also, women who get married earlier are unable to complete their higher education, which is imperative for professional stability and specialized recruitment. Child marriage is sustained by culture, religious interpretation, and the dominance of traditional laws over state laws, leading to numerous health problems such as physical deficiencies for the mother, deformity in the child, risk of disease in adult years of the child, and risk of maternal and child mortality.

Medicine and healthcare for women are not only about health recovery and well-being but also mainly about exercising control over women; this control may be yielded by neocolonialist interests to control the population and resources of South Asia or by indigenous patriarchal forces (Ginsburg and Rapp 1991). Many women in South Asia have suffered health consequences of sterilization and birth control policies, such as infertility, hormonal imbalances, gynaecological problems, and other disabling side effects (Hartmann 1995). It is mostly the disadvantaged and marginalized women groups that have become susceptible to sterilization and birth control campaigns due to payment and subsidization in cash by vested agents. A classic example of successful civilian resistance against unfair health policies is the mass riots in India held against the national sterilization campaign of the 1970s. As the patriarchal order was threatened, the men were able to overturn the campaign. However, when unfair or political policies for women's health are promoted, there is less of a cultural backlash from men in South Asia. Thus, it is suggested that in the case of state sponsorship for campaigns that place women's health at risk, it is men that must be relied upon to become the greatest champions for women's equality and development.

8.9 Recommendations for Health Policy Protection of Women

Dependency on foreign agencies and NGOs is not a long-term or holistic solution for women's health needs in South Asia. Needless to say, there needs to be indigenous, systematic, and long-term public health policy implementation in the region. The principals of gender equity have to become conditions for the regional development of women's health under three broad areas of health improvement, health protection, and health services. The developed world has to succeed in improving general health statistics for women, and many of their policies and programmes must be considered for improvement in South Asia. However, there is a problem with rigid benchmarking and emulation of health policies for women, in that if they are not planned in consideration of regional socio-economic realities and cultural traditions, they may not be as effective in South Asia. What works for Singapore in terms of health financing may not work in South Asia due to population differences, and similarly, what may work in Sweden with regard to family planning policies may not work in South Asia due to differences in preferences for family size. Thus, there is need for a focused and indigenous public health policy for the holistic development of South Asian women's health quality of life. Table 8.1 summarizes the initiatives that the state must take to secure women's health and overall development in South Asia.

8.9.1 Public Healthcare Services

A pressing need for the public health sector of South Asia is to deliver quality services from primary to the tertiary sector and to fulfil a continuum of care across the life course of women. There also needs to be emergency preparedness especially in lieu of regional conflict and high numbers of girl and women refugees, internally displaced persons (IDPs), and widowed women in the country. The quality of public healthcare services must be secured through third-party monitoring of service provision and the integration of ministries, such as the health ministry, women's ministry, the social welfare ministry, and the population ministry. There needs to be state sponsorship for all-encompassing community-based initiatives for women's health including: (i) complaint cells, (ii) women health committees, and (iii) third-party monitoring bodies.

There is a need for consistent public audits exclusively for women in order to get feedback about women's health services. In addition, what is important is that for valid and reliable feedback, women must be aware of their basic health rights, human rights, and political citizenship rights. So if there are community programmes for women's health audits, they should be coupled first with awareness about needs and rights. Perhaps, in bureaucracies like that of South Asia, where corruption and inefficiency are rampant, the placement of health ombudsmen across community spaces must be introduced to report instances of practitioner license, practitioner violations of code of conduct, pharmaceutical violations, and centre violations.

Table 8.1 Target recommendations for government public policy for women's health in South Asia[a]

1. Public healthcare services	2. Access for all women populations	3. Participation of women across structures	4. Wider social policies for women	5. Specific health policies for women	6. State licensing and regulation	7. Public health laws	8. Government health budget
Quality of healthcare services	Rural areas	Political participation	Poverty alleviation	Gender screening and gender selection	Healthcare practitioners	Women's health statistics database	Health practitioner institutes
Primary to tertiary sector services	Marginalized populations	Women's employment in the formal sector of economy	Compulsory enrolment and retention in the education sector	Birth spacing and family planning	Complementary and alternative medicine	Communicable disease, preventable healthcare, and toxic exposure	Compensation and benefits of practitioners
Continuum of care	Awareness of health needs and health services	Increase in women health workers	Workplace laws and employment benefits	Prenatal and postnatal assistance from trained practitioners and institutional delivery	Pharmaceutical industry	Vaccination and immunization	Resources and medical equipment
Emergency preparedness	Cultural acceptance	Gender quotas in public offices, parliament, and private organizations	Marriage age and divorce rights	Food safety and nutritional supplementation	Illicit drug and tobacco control	School healthcare	Ratios of hospital beds to patients
Community healthcare services	Health financing	Sports and leisure activities	Subsidies for women families[a]	Domestic violence and corporal punishment screening in hospitals and schools		Air pollution	
	Use of technology		Mental health	Reproductive health		Clean household energy supply	

[a]Data in this table has been compiled by the authors

8.9.2 Access for All Women Populations

Though urban and elite women face fewer problems, majority of women in South Asia from rural and remote areas need special consideration for healthcare services. Marginalized populations from the interiors, villages, and mountainous areas require combined federal and provincial health protection. There is also need to address the health needs of other hidden populations like the third gender, the disabled, and ageing women. The awareness of health needs and services in women populations, the illiterate, semi-literate, and impoverished, is also critical. There needs to be cultural acceptance for trained medical practitioners and seeking of healthcare services for women in the region.

Both universal health protection and employee health protection schemes need to be introduced and improved in South Asia to ensure that unprivileged women are able to access services without fear of indebtedness or bankruptcy. Technology can become an important tool for two diverse purposes: (i) to help the masses and remote populations become aware of prevention and health services, and (ii) to help keep better records of health history for the continuum of care. In order to promote women's health, the governments of South Asia need to take a more holistic social policy approach by improving culture and traditions through the use of media, religious authorities, and community notables.

8.9.3 Participation of Women Across Structures

South Asian women are critically underrepresented across key structures of society which could afford them opportunities for health advancement. Improving women's political participation and awareness of citizenship rights is the first step to improving women's health. Participation of women in all three sectors of politics, the formal sector of the economy, and the health sector is imperative for women-driven improvements in health and the overall development for women. Gender quotas in public offices, parliament, and private organizations are necessary. In addition, quotas for marginalized populations based on ethnicity and disability must further have gender-based conditions, as marginalized and disabled women are not provided equal opportunities in both public and private sectors compared to the men. The promotion of sports and leisure activities in women would be beneficial in reducing the health burden and improving the health quality of lives overall, as physical activities should no longer be retained for men in the region.

8.9.4 Wider Social Policies for Women

Improvements in women's health are not possible unless a comprehensive approach is adopted by the governments of South Asia with regard to social policy. Prudent and longitudinal policies for poverty alleviation, compulsory enrolment and retention in the education sector, workplace laws, marriage age and divorce rights, mental health, and sports and leisure activities are needed. Employment benefits for women must include minimum wages, paternal leave, maternal benefits, paid leave, pension and provident funds, lactation and day-care centres, options for home-based employment, and security against dismissal during maternal leave.

State subsidization mechanisms can assist in increasing social support and cultural acceptance for the girl child. Subsidies for the following groups is essential: (i) families with daughters, (ii) single women running a household (with dependents like ageing parents, younger siblings, niece, or nephews), (iii) single mothers (divorced, separated, and widowed), (iv) women who are unemployed or in the informal sector of the economy, and (v) ageing women.

8.9.5 Specific Health Policies for Women

Research shows that when fair laws for gender and health are enforced, there is an association with improved health indicators for women including maternal mortality (Pinzon-Rondon et al. 2015). However, more specific health policies for the women of South Asia are also needed. The South Asian region is in dire need of policies to prevent gender screening and gender selection to prevent female foeticide. Birth spacing and family planning, prenatal and postnatal assistance from trained practitioners, and institutional deliveries would help to reduce maternal and child mortality rates. Public sector hospitals in South Asia must have policies to screen for domestic violence of wives or corporal punishment of daughters. There is also immediate need for food safety and nutritional access for women, including nutritional supplementation, as women are comparatively more undernourished in the region compared to men. Gathering of longitudinal data about comparative nutrition and stunting between males and females is also needed.

8.9.6 State Licensing and Regulation

The lack of licensing and regulation has become a major impediment for women's health outcomes in South Asia. Four areas need to be strictly licensed and regulated by South Asian governments, which are: (i) healthcare practitioners, (ii) complementary and alternative medicine providers, (iii) the pharmaceutical industry, and (iv) illicit drug and tobacco usage. The expansion of a regulation and licensing sector will also help create jobs and reduce unemployment in South Asia. Better regulation and compensation will also help to reduce the brain drain of qualified healthcare practitioners and strengthen the health workforce in order to improve patient safety and public health standards.

8.9.7 Public Health Laws

Discussion from this chapter indicates that public health laws are not comprehensive or enacted in South Asia. The modern world laissez-faire ethic and free market dynamics are used as justification for neglect of the reformation of public health laws. There is also concern that public health laws can be used as a political tool to control and manipulate populations. With geopolitical conflict and foreign intervention in some parts of South Asia, there is the additional fear that public health laws could be misused by external agents to manipulate social change. Public health laws of South Asia need to be introduced or reformed, specifically with regard to: (1) women's health statistics, (2) communicable disease, preventable health care, and toxic exposure, (3) vaccination and immunization, (4) school health care, (5) air pollution, (6) clean household energy supply, and (7) water supply and infrastructure.

8.9.8 Government Health Budget

The government budgets in South Asia need to be significantly increased in order to improve healthcare training institutes, compensation and benefits of practitioners, resources and medical equipment, and staffing or ratios of health services to patients. Once the organizational culture is not characteristic of resource and practitioner shortage, there will be an increase in recruitment and retention of practitioners in the region and the consequent improvement in patient mortality and morbidity.

References

Ahmed, N., Deshpande, S., Feruglio, F., & Nisbett, N. (2016). *Accountability in health and nutrition in South Asia–A conceptual and practical review of lessons from the global literature and from India, Pakistan and Bangladesh*. Institute of Development Studies: Falmer.

Akhtar, S., Ismail, T., Atukorala, S., & Arlappa, N. (2013). Micronutrient deficiencies in South Asia–Current status and strategies. *Trends in Food Science & Technology, 31*(1), 55–62.

Angell, M., & Kassirer, J. P. (1998). *Alternative medicine – The risks of untested and unregulated remedies*. Waltham: Massachusetts Medical Society.

Annandale, E. (2005). Gender and health status: Does biology matter? In *Debating biology* (pp. 94–105). London: Routledge.

Annandale, E. (2008). *Women's health and social change*. New York: Routledge.

Asian Development Bank. (2018). *Key indicators for Asia and the Pacific 2018*. Retrieved from https://www.adb.org/sites/default/files/publication/443671/ki2018.pdf

Azhar, S., Hassali, M. A., Ibrahim, M. I. M., Ahmad, M., Masood, I., & Shafie, A. A. (2009). The role of pharmacists in developing countries: The current scenario in Pakistan. *Journal of Health and Human Resources Administration, 7*(1), 54.

Bambra, C., Fox, D., & Scott-Samuel, A. (2005). Towards a politics of health. *Health Promotion International, 20*(2), 187–193.

Basu, S., Andrews, J., Kishore, S., Panjabi, R., & Stuckler, D. (2012). Comparative performance of private and public healthcare systems in low-and middle-income countries: A systematic review. *PLoS Medicine, 9*(6), e1001244.

Baxter, C. (2002). *Government and politics in South Asia*. Boulder: Westview Press.

Beasley, A., & Amir, L. H. (2007). *Infant feeding, poverty and human development*. London: BioMed Central.

Begum, F. S. (2016). *Gender equality and women's empowerment: Suggested strategies for the 7th five year plan*. Dhaka: General Economics Division: Planning Commission of Government Bangladesh. Accessed, 8.

Benn, T., Pfister, G., & Jawad, H. (2010). *Muslim women and sport*. London: Routledge.

Berro Pizzarossa, L. (2018). Here to stay: The evolution of sexual and reproductive health and rights in International Human Rights Law. *Laws, 7*(3), 29.

Bezbaruah, S. (2012). *Gender inequalities in India's new service economy: A case study of the banking sector.*

Bhatia, K. (2014). Community health worker programs in India: A rights-based review. *Perspectives in Public Health, 134*(5), 276–282.

Bhutta, Z. A., Gupta, I., de'Silva, H., Manandhar, D., Awasthi, S., Hossain, S. M., & Salam, M. (2004). Maternal and child health: Is South Asia ready for change? *BMJ, 328*(7443), 816–819.

Blair, R. D., & Durrance, C. P. (2014). Licensing health care professionals, state action and anti-trust policy. *Iowa Law Review, 100*, 1943.

Bodeker, G., & Ong, C.-K. (2005). *WHO global atlas of traditional, complementary and alternative medicine* (Vol. 1). Geneva: World Health Organization.

Brhlikova, P., Harper, I., Jeffery, R., Rawal, N., Subedi, M., & Santhosh, M. (2011). Trust and the regulation of pharmaceuticals: South Asia in a globalised world. *Globalization and Health, 7*(1), 10.

Carroll, A. E. (2017). The high costs of unnecessary care. *JAMA, 318*(18), 1748–1749.

Chakraborty, L. (2016). *Asia: A survey of gender budgeting efforts*. Washington, DC: International Monetary Fund.

Chakravarthi, I. (2013). Medical equipment industry in India: Production, procurement and utilization. *Indian Journal of Public Health, 57*(4), 203.

Chopra, A., Saluja, M., Tillu, G., Sarmukkaddam, S., Venugopalan, A., Narsimulu, G., et al. (2013). Ayurvedic medicine offers a good alternative to glucosamine and celecoxib in the treatment of symptomatic knee osteoarthritis: A randomized, double-blind, controlled equivalence drug trial. *The Journal of Rheumatology, 52*(8), 1408–1417.

Cnattingius, S. (2004). The epidemiology of smoking during pregnancy: Smoking prevalence, maternal characteristics, and pregnancy outcomes. *Nicotine & Tobacco Research, 6*(Suppl_2), S125–S140.

Das, S., Alcock, G., Azad, K., Kuddus, A., Manandhar, D. S., Shrestha, B. P., et al. (2016). Institutional delivery in public and private sectors in South Asia: A comparative analysis of prospective data from four demographic surveillance sites. *BMC Pregnancy and Childbirth, 16*(1), 273.

Dasvarma, G. (2003). Population and environmental issues in South Asia. In *South Asia* (p. 35). New York: Routledge – Taylor and Francis Group.

Drugs, U. N. O. O., & Crime. (2010). *World drug report 2010*. New York: United Nations Publications.

Dyson, T. (2012). Causes and consequences of skewed sex ratios. *Annual Review of Sociology, 38*, 443–461.
Economakis, G., Rizopoulos, Y., & Sergakis, D. (2010). Patterns of corruption. *Journal of Economics and Business, 13*(2), 11–31.
El-Saharty, S., Chowdhury, S., Ohno, N., & Sarker, I. (2016). *Improving maternal and reproductive health in South Asia: Drivers and enablers*. Washington, DC: The World Bank.
Engelgau, M. M., El-Saharty, S., Kudesia, P., Rajan, V., Rosenhouse, S., & Okamoto, K. (2011). *Capitalizing on the demographic transition: Tackling noncommunicable diseases in South Asia*. Washington, DC: The World Bank.
Filmer, D., & King, E. (1999). *Gender disparity in South Asia: Comparisons between and within countries*. Washington, DC: The World Bank.
Friedman, S. H., & Resnick, P. J. (2007). Child murder by mothers: Patterns and prevention. *World Psychiatry, 6*(3), 137.
Garnweidner, L. M., Terragni, L., Pettersen, K. S., & Mosdøl, A. (2012). Perceptions of the host country's food culture among female immigrants from Africa and Asia: Aspects relevant for cultural sensitivity in nutrition communication. *Journal of Nutrition Education and Behavior, 44*(4), 335–342.
Ghaffar, A., Reddy, K. S., & Singhi, M. (2004). Burden of non-communicable diseases in South Asia. *BMJ: British Medical Journal, 328*(7443), 807.
Ginsburg, F., & Rapp, R. (1991). The politics of reproduction. *Annual Review of Anthropology, 20*(1), 311–343.
Golshan, A., Patel, C., & Hyder, A. A. (2013). A systematic review of the epidemiology of unintentional burn injuries in South Asia. *Journal of Public Health, 35*(3), 384–396.
Goonesekere, S. (2004). *Violence, law and women's rights in South Asia*. New Delhi: SAGE Publications.
Gupta, M. D. (2005). Explaining Asia's "missing women": A new look at the data. *Population and Development Review, 31*(3), 529–535.
Haatanen, M. (2015). *The effects of medicalization, medical practices, and mental disorder on the subjective experience of the self in Sarah Kane's 4.48 psychosis*.
Haque, M. S. (2003). Reinventing governance for performance in South Asia: Impacts on citizenship rights. *International Journal of Public Administration, 26*(8–9), 941–964.
Hartmann, B. (1995). *Reproductive rights and wrongs: The global politics of population control*. Boston: South End Press.
Hazarika, G. (2000). Gender differences in children's nutrition and access to health care in Pakistan. *The Journal of Development Studies, 37*(1), 73–92.
Hunt, J., & Kasynathan, N. (2001). Pathways to empowerment? Reflections on microfinance and transformation in gender relations in South Asia. *Gender and Development, 9*(1), 42–52.
Islam, A., & Biswas, T. (2014). Health system in Bangladesh: Challenges and opportunities. *American Journal of Health Research, 2*(6), 366–374.
Iwanaga, K. (2008). *Women's political participation and representation in Asia: Obstacles and challenges*. Copenhagen: NIAS Press.
Jafree, S. R. (2018). *Women, healthcare, and violence in Pakistan*. Karachi: Oxford University Press.
Janoski, T., Alford, R. R., Hicks, A. M., & Schwartz, M. A. (2005). *The handbook of political sociology: States, civil societies, and globalization*. New York: Cambridge University Press.
Kandiyoti, D. (1988). Bargaining with patriarchy. *Gender & Society, 2*(3), 274–290.
Kane, P., Dennerstein, L., & Organization, W. H. (1999). Women and occupational health: Issues and policy paper for the Global Commission on Women's Health/editor: Penny Kane; project director: Lorraine Dennerstein. In *Women and occupational health: issues and policy paper for the Global Commission on Women's Health/editor: Penny Kane; project director: Lorraine Dennerstein*.
Kastor, A., & Mohanty, S. K. (2018). Disease-specific out-of-pocket and catastrophic health expenditure on hospitalization in India: Do Indian households face distress health financing? *PLoS One, 13*(5), e0196106.

Kelkar, G. (2007). *The feminization of agriculture in Asia: Implications for women's agency and productivity*. Taipei: ASPAC Food & Fertilizer Technology Center.
Kensy, J., Stengal, C., Nougier, M., & Birgin, R. (2012). *Drug policy and women: Addressing the negative consequences of harmful drug control*. London: International Drug Policy Consortium.
Klasen, S., & Wink, C. (2003). "Missing women": Revisiting the debate. *Feminist Economics, 9*(2–3), 263–299.
Kramlich, D. (2014). Introduction to complementary, alternative, and traditional therapies. *Critical Care Nurse, 34*(6), 50–56.
Krishna, B., Balakrishnan, K., Siddiqui, A. R., Begum, B. A., Bachani, D., & Brauer, M. (2017). Tackling the health burden of air pollution in South Asia. *BMJ, 359*, j5209.
Krook, M. L., & Norris, P. (2014). Beyond quotas: Strategies to promote gender equality in elected office. *Political Studies, 62*(1), 2–20.
Kuhn, S., Milasi, S., & Yoon, S. (2018). *World employment social outlook: Trends 2018*. Geneva: ILO.
Kumari, S., & Singh, A. K. (2016). Working women in informal sector: Geographical perspective. *Journal of the Anthropological Survey of India, 65*(2), 185–199.
Lafferty, A., Treacy, M. P., Fealy, G., Drennan, J., & Lyons, I. (2012). *Older people's experiences of mistreatment and abuse*. Dublin: NCPOP, University College Dublin.
Larson, J. S. (1999). The conceptualization of health. *Medical Care Research and Review, 56*(2), 123–136.
Latten, T., Westra, D., Angeli, F., Paulus, A., Struss, M., & Ruwaard, D. (2018). Pharmaceutical companies and healthcare providers: Going beyond the gift–An explorative review. *PLoS One, 13*(2), e0191856.
Lewis, M. (2006). *Governance and corruption in public health care systems*. Washington, DC: Centre for Global Development.
Light, D. W. (2007). Professional dominance in medicine. In *The Blackwell encyclopedia of sociology* (pp. 1–5). New York: Blackwell.
Low, W.-Y., Lee, Y.-K., & Samy, A. L. (2015). Non-communicable diseases in the Asia-Pacific region: Prevalence, risk factors and community-based prevention. *International Journal of Occupational Medicine and Environmental Health, 28*, 1–7.
Maestre, M., & Poole, N. (2018). Value chains for nutrition in South Asia: Who delivers, how, and to whom? *IDS Bulletin, 49*, 1–20.
Maghsoudlou, S., Cnattingius, S., Montgomery, S., Aarabi, M., Semnani, S., Wikström, A.-K., & Bahmanyar, S. (2018). Opium use during pregnancy and infant size at birth: A cohort study. *BMC Pregnancy and Childbirth, 18*(1), 358.
Maitra, B., & Mukhopadhyay, C. K. (2012). Public spending on education, health care and economic growth in selected countries of Asia and the Pacific. *Pacific Development Journal, 19*(2), 19–48.
Marphatia, A. A., Ambale, G. S., & Reid, A. M. (2017). Women's marriage age matters for public health: A review of the broader health and social implications in South Asia. *Frontiers in Public Health, 5*, 269.
Md Illias Kanchan, Firoz, M., Anand, A., & Biswas, A. B. (2017). Utilization of skilled birth attendant in South Asian region: A comparative study of India, Bangladesh and Nepal. *European Journal of Pharmaceutical and Medical Research, 4*(10), 305–311.
Misau, Y. A., Al-Sadat, N., & Gerei, A. B. (2010). Brain-drain and health care delivery in developing countries. *Journal of Public Health in Africa, 1*(1), e6.
Mishra, V., Roy, T. K., & Retherford, R. D. (2004). Sex differentials in childhood feeding, health care, and nutritional status in India. *Population and Development Review, 30*(2), 269–295.
Misra, A., Khurana, L., Isharwal, S., & Bhardwaj, S. (2008). South Asian diets and insulin resistance. *British Journal of Nutrition, 101*(4), 465–473.
Morgan, R., & Ensor, T. (2016). The regulation of private hospitals in Asia. *The International Journal of Health Planning and Management, 31*(1), 49–64.

Müller, O., & Krawinkel, M. (2005). Malnutrition and health in developing countries. *CMAJ, 173*(3), 279–286.
Nanayakkara, S. (2012). Crossing boundaries and changing identities: Empowering South Asian women through sport and physical activities. *The International Journal of the History of Sport, 29*(13), 1885–1906.
Nash, J. C., & Fernández-Kelly, M. P. (1983). *Women, men, and the international division of labor*. New York: Suny Press.
Niaz, U. (2003). Violence against women in South Asian countries. *Archives of Women's Mental Health, 6*(3), 173–184.
Omvedt, G. (2005). Women in governance in South Asia. *Economic and Political Weekly, 40*, 4746–4752.
Organization, W. H. (2007). *Women, ageing and health: A framework for action: Focus on gender*. Geneva: WHO.
Organization, W. H. (2014). *Injuries and violence: The facts 2014*. Geneva: World Health Organization.
Osman, F. A. (2008). Health policy, programmes and system in Bangladesh: Achievements and challenges. *South Asian Survey, 15*(2), 263–288.
Osmani, S., & Sen, A. (2003). The hidden penalties of gender inequality: Fetal origins of ill-health. *Economics & Human Biology, 1*(1), 105–121.
Pallas, S. W., Minhas, D., Pérez-Escamilla, R., Taylor, L., Curry, L., & Bradley, E. H. (2013). Community health workers in low-and middle-income countries: What do we know about scaling up and sustainability? *American Journal of Public Health, 103*(7), e74–e82.
Pinzon-Rondon, A. M., Attaran, A., Botero, J. C., & Ruiz-Sternberg, A. M. (2015). Association of rule of law and health outcomes: An ecological study. *BMJ Open, 5*(10), e007004.
Porter, D. (2005). *Health, civilization and the state: A history of public health from ancient to modern times*. New York: Routledge.
Price, G., Alam, R., Hasan, S., Humayun, F., Kabir, M., Karki, C., et al. (2014). *Attitudes to water in South Asia*. London: Royal Institute of International Affairs.
Punjani, N. S., Shams, S., & Bhanji, S. M. (2014). Analysis of health care delivery systems: Pakistan versus United States. *International Journal of Endorsing Health Science Research, 2*(1), 38–41.
Qureshi, K. (2017). *Ageing: Gender, social class and health in Pakistan*. In: Retrieved February.
Rai, S. M., Bari, F., Mahtab, N., & Mohanty, B. (2006). South Asia: Gender quotas and the politics of empowerment–A comparative study. In D. Dahlerup (Ed.), *Women, quotas and politics* (pp. 222–245). New York: Routledge.
Raj, A., McDougal, L., & Rusch, M. L. (2012). Changes in prevalence of girl child marriage in South Asia. *JAMA, 307*(19), 2027–2029.
Ray, R., Kattimani, S., & Sharma, H. (2006). *Opium abuse and its management: Global scenario* (pp. 1–13). New Delhi: World Health Organization Department of Mental Health and Substance Abuse Management of Substance Abuse. National Drug Dependence Treatment Centre All India Institute of Medical Sciences.
Reid, C., Dyck, L., McKay, H., & Frisby, W. (2005). The health benefits of physical activity for girls and women. *Centres of Excellence for Women's Health Research Bulletin, 4*(2), 10.
Roberts, M., Hsiao, W., Berman, P., & Reich, M. (2003). *Getting health reform right: A guide to improving performance and equity*. Oxford/New York: Oxford University Press.
Sassen-Koob, S. (1983). Labor migrations and the new international division of labor. In *Women, men and the International Division of Labor* (pp. 175–204). Albany: State University of New York Press.
Scheper-Hughes, N., Alter, J. S., Ayora-Diaz, S. I., Csordas, T. J., Frankenburg, R., Leyton, E., et al. (2000). The global traffic in human organs. *Current Anthropology, 41*(2), 191–224.
Sheykhi, M. T. (2007). Ageing and quality of life in Asia and Europe: A comparative sociological appraisal. In *Quality of life in old age* (pp. 167–177). Dordrecht: Springer.

Shrivastava, S. R., Shrivastava, P. S., & Ramasamy, J. (2015). Mainstreaming of Ayurveda, Yoga, Naturopathy, Unani, Siddha, and Homeopathy with the health care delivery system in India. *Journal of Traditional and Complementary Medicine, 5*(2), 116–118.

Sudha, S., & Rajan, S. I. (1999). Female demographic disadvantage in India 1981–1991: Sex selective abortions and female infanticide. *Development and Change, 30*(3), 585–618.

Swaminathan, S., Qureshi, H., Jahan, M. U., Baskota, D. K., De Alwis, S., & Dandona, L. (2017). Health research priorities and gaps in South Asia. *BMJ, 357*, j1510.

Thomas, M., & Thomas, M. (2002). *Status of women with disabilities in South Asia* (Selected readings in community-based rehabilitation, series, 2). Bangalore: APDRJ.

Tiwari, R., Negandhi, H., & Zodpey, S. P. (2018). Health management workforce for India in 2030. *Frontiers in Public Health, 6*, 227.

Tong, R. (1998). The ethics of care: A feminist virtue ethics of care for healthcare practitioners. *The Journal of Medicine and Philosophy, 23*(2), 131–152.

United Nations. (2010). *The World's women 2010: Trends and statistics*. New York: UN.

United Nations- Economic and Social Commission for Asia and the Pacific. (2007). *Harmful traditional practices in three countries of South Asia: Culture, human rights and violence against women* (Gender and development discussion paper series, 21). United Nations- Economic and Social Commission for Asia and the Pacific: Bangkok.

van Weel, C., Kassai, R., Qidwai, W., Kumar, R., Bala, K., Gupta, P. P., et al. (2016). Primary healthcare policy implementation in South Asia. *BMJ Global Health, 1*(2), e000057.

Vergne, C. (2009). Democracy, elections and allocation of public expenditures in developing countries. *European Journal of Political Economy, 25*(1), 63–77.

Waylen, G. (2005). Analysing women in the politics of the Third World. In *Women and politics in the Third World* (pp. 20–37). London: Routledge.

Wellalage, N., & Locke, S. (2017). Access to credit by SMEs in South Asia: Do women entrepreneurs face discrimination. *Research in International Business and Finance, 41*, 336–346.

World Bank Group. (2014). *World development indicators 2014*. Washington, DC: World Bank Publications.

World Economic Forum. (2017). *The global gender gap report 2017*. Retrieved from http://www3.weforum.org/docs/WEF_GGGR_2017.pdf

World Health Organization. (2018). *World health statistics 2018: Monitoring health for the Sustainable Development Goals*. Geneva: World Health Organization.

Yaya, S., Bishwajit, G., & Ekholuenetale, M. (2017). Factors associated with the utilization of institutional delivery services in Bangladesh. *PLoS One, 12*(2), e0171573.

Yazbeck, A. S., & Peters, D. H. (2003). *Health policy research in South Asia: Building capacity for reform*. Washington, DC: The World Bank.

Zaidi, S., Saligram, P., Ahmed, S., Sonderp, E., & Sheikh, K. (2017). Expanding access to healthcare in South Asia. *BMJ, 357*, j1645.

Ziltener, P., & Künzler, D. (2013). Impacts of colonialism—A research survey. *Journal of World-Systems Research, 19*(2), 290–311.

Chapter 9
The Culture of Health Regulation and Its Implications on Maternal and Reproductive Health in South Asia

Ainul Momina and Sara Rizvi Jafree

9.1 Introduction

We have already established two important matters so far in this book, with regard to improving healthcare support for women: firstly, that state intervention is imperative to improve women's health behaviour and health outcomes and, secondly, that maternal and reproductive health services have been prioritized over all other health services in South Asia. In this chapter, we intend to discuss optimal health regulatory practices, in context to functioning maternal health services. There is no doubt that culture and traditions influence regulatory practices of the state, and in fact, it is culture that is responsible for sustaining regressive and inefficient regulatory policies in a nation (Cleary et al. 2013;Manville et al. 2013). We believe it is imperative to try and change this culture of abandonment and propose a better regulatory health framework for South Asia, in order to improve health services and protection of women. We hope this work will help to map policies for improvement in maternal health, given higher mortality in South Asia, and also help develop plans for other healthcare services for women in the region. Regulation is the sustained and focused control exercised by a public agency over activities that are valued by a community (Walshe 2003). It is suggested that regulation is established as a continuous activity with a clear direction, firmly rooted in the public sector with public interest as the main goal and where only public institutions are responsible for regulation.

The critical role of the state in regulating and facilitating the overall management of a diverse and demanding health sector in developing countries has come under renewed focus. Realization has dawned that health care is a risky business. Analysis

A. Momina (✉)
King Edward Medical University, Lahore, Pakistan

S. R. Jafree
Department of Sociology, Forman Christian College University, Lahore, Pakistan

S. R. Jafree (ed.), *The Sociology of South Asian Women's Health*,
https://doi.org/10.1007/978-3-030-50204-1_9

of credible data revealed that over 10% of patients experience some type of adverse event in hospitals or at health facilities (Webb et al. 1993). In South Asia, the situation is even direr, with regard to unfavourable error reporting, low patient safety, and adverse health outcomes, especially for women and children (Chakravarty et al. 2015;Jafree et al. 2015). Estimates and consensus from other countries suggest that a large proportion of errors are preventable. The challenge for safety and quality is to design safer systems and inculcate a culture of safety (Sheikh et al. 2013), and the challenge for governance essentially is to ensure that these systems and practices are applied in reality (Healy and Braithwaite 2006). Multifarious reasons are attributed for the challenges encountered in health regulation which will be discussed in detail subsequently. At the outset, it is important to note that the extensive and ever-expansive size of the private sector involvement has led to marketization of the health sector. This requires a strengthened role of the state (Kumaranayake and Watts 2000). The catch, however, lies in the fact that limiting the regulatory effort in the health sector to the state alone has implications for the success and robustness of the effort and outcomes. This is especially true for a region like South Asia, where state policies and regulatory efforts are influenced by regressive gender-based values. To take an example, the Jirga laws and feudal system have more control over the practices of women for health care as opposed to state laws. And this is what we need to discern at various levels.

9.2 Types of Regulation by State

When it comes to regulation of the health sector, the traditional focus has been a standard setting, as in the shape and form of ensuring minimum levels of quality and safety. This approach often termed as "social," can be distinguished from the more "economic" approach, which looks at the role of regulation in the context of markets (Ogus 1996). However, the "social" approach must be extended to consider the cultural commitment to ensuring quality, safety, and equity in health services. Definitions presenting a social focus emphasize control, public authority, and the power of the state; emphasize using regulatory instruments of a bureaucratic nature; and require state authority to enforce regulations or influence behaviour in tangible terms (Baldwin et al. 1999). Social control is premised to include regulation in a way that emphasizes social cohesion, equity, and protection as an aim. What is explicit is that "command" and "deliberate state of influence" are usually understood to be state functions. At the core of health regulation lies the aim of changing individual and organizational behaviour in health care, essentially through the use of coercive power (Roberts et al. 2004). Regulatory instruments and legal tools are applied through the state apparatus. Little scope is allowed for negotiation amongst different actors, and the state is perceived as the dominant regulatory authority.

Another school of thought defines regulation in an economic context as government controlling or deliberately trying to influence the activities of actors by manipulating such variables as price, quantity, and quality (Kumaranayake and Watts

2000). The responsibility rests firmly with state authorities, and it is assumed that manipulation of market rules for price, quantity, and quality is sufficient to influence the behaviour of market actors and can lead to economic efficiency. Measurement of these variables would require considerable market behaviour and outcome data that are seldom available in developing countries. Attention has, therefore, tended to focus on quantity and quality controls amongst regulators in developing countries (Kadaï et al. 2006).

Mackintosh focuses solely on the commercial sector and introduces the private health insurance industry in the discourse for health regulation (Mackintosh 2007). Regulation from this context is defined as actions by the state regulatory agencies to influence the private sector to provide health services and health insurance through market sale and with objectives of profit. Actions needed to fulfil this mandate include price-setting rules, standards, competition policies, restrictions on the organizational forms of market actors, and consumer rights licenses. Qualified providers are mostly not accessible or affordable by the poor, who in turn rely on private informal providers that are largely unregulated. This is especially a problem in South Asia, given high poverty levels and the feminization of poverty specifically. Current systems of regulation in developing countries are unable to control private healthcare systems in earnest. One salient reason for this is a lack of information or knowledge on the behaviour and activities of commercial, particularly informal providers (Bloom et al. 2009).

There is also the "Command and Control" view, in which the state calls the shots as it is in the driving seat (Aalders and Wilthagen 1997). The state usually invokes legal and punitive power. It is documented to be a mostly non-inclusive and top-down regulatory system. One example is immediate and fair punitive actions against illegal reproductive health clinics and abortion centres in South Asia. The government is perceived as the single driver behind regulation, selectively deploying and adjusting these actions as per situation and ground reality. A major concern of this form of regulation is the equity of access, especially in developing countries and countries that have patriarchal states which neglect women. Currently, the health sector of South Asia is characterized by intricacies of variegated nature, complexity, a plurality of players and multitude stakeholders, rapid change in its environment, and a recent proliferation of regulatory strategies. This is why a one-size-fits-all solution is not likely to work in a sector as complex as health for South Asia.

9.3 Challenges to Effective Regulation in South Asia

Medical negligence is rife in developing countries. However, under-reporting is also a matter of serious concern. Under-reporting of medical negligence is influenced by the inadequate culture of patient safety, lack of knowledge in patients, and the absence of accountability against perpetrators (Raposo 2015;Jafree 2018). Medical negligence is undisputedly a mandate of regulation. Due to systemic shortcomings primarily, the medical negligence cases end up with police taking cognizance, with very little capacity to understand and prosecute (Jawaid 2014). A review of the literature identifies constraints on effective systems for regulation of the commercial health sector in developing countries, including poor enforcement, limited institutional capacity, and cost-effectiveness of regulations (Brhlikova et al. 2011). Whilst being a generic problem, this assumes serious proportions when it comes to regulation, since health regulation requires a skill set of a higher order. Minimum Service Delivery Standards (MSDS) requires the availability of a specified number of trained human resources, whilst South Asia is a region that faces a health workforce crisis (WHO 2006). Local studies have asserted that hiring qualified ancillary staff and maintaining clinics according to MSDS requires not only investing more capital but also raising the overheads manifold (Momina et al. 2016).

Poor enforcement of health regulation is reported as a primary problem (Ensor and Weinzierl 2007). The administrative burden of bureaucratic approaches to regulation can be considerable (Teerawattananon et al. 2003). Regulation requires adequate monitoring and information systems and mechanisms for decision-making about violations and guidelines on when and how to apply sanctions. For these reasons, failure to enforce regulation is usually attributed to lack of institutional capacity (WHO 2000). The impact of competing priorities is also an important reason that regulation may not be enforced. An empirical study that examined the enforcement of pharmaceutical regulations in a developing country revealed that the licensing of facilities had been introduced, but regulators had not developed sanctions in case of violations (Stenson et al. 2001). Moreover, due to lack of resources, trade-offs had to be made with the geographical distribution of pharmacies and enforcing quality regulation.

Regulation and enforcement are dependent on institutional capacity, which is generally weaker in low-income countries than in middle-income countries (WHO 2000). Middle-income countries may have much larger commercial health sectors, as well as more resources to channel into regulation. Findings from regulation studies in other developing countries like Zimbabwe, Tanzania (Kumaranayake 2000), Laos (Stenson 1997) and Thailand (Teerawattananon et al. 2003) illustrate these differences. In Thailand, roles and responsibilities of regulators and regulations that covered both public and private sectors were found to be comprehensive. Administrative structures, rules, incentives, and standards were firmly in place, indicating that Thailand had reached a stage of institutional development and capacity that can produce these regulatory systems. However, low-income countries, including states in South Asia, had not accomplished these, mostly due to the lack of institutional development and the limited availability of resources. This critical and fundamental difference between countries cannot be ignored.

Compared to middle-income countries, in low-income countries, there are more international actors, including NGOs, UN agencies, and bilateral donors. They provide resources and exert influence on health policy, strategy, and implementation (Palmer et al. 2006). The distinction between countries with low or virtually nonexistent institutional capacity and those with more developed institutional capacity determines the capacity level at which analysis for regulatory reform begins. Experience shows that if regulatory frameworks are adopted at the right time, the worst problems may be avoided or at least managed, but once the private sector has grown large, it is difficult to introduce regulation (Kumaranayake 1997; Mills et al. 2002). This is actually happening in almost all of the South Asian countries, in particular, the ones with large populations like India and Pakistan.

In developing countries, regulation generally focuses on formal-sector commercial providers through licensing of health professionals, pharmaceuticals, medical technologies, and health facilities. Defining standards for performance, such as through the accreditation of hospitals, is a more common practice but is considered more of a voluntary bargain (Ensor and Weinzierl 2007). Regulation becomes a pressing need if the behaviour of commercial sector providers is seen to be undermining or in contradiction with national health goals. The example of managing infectious diseases like dengue and more recently coronavirus is a case in point. South Asian governments stepped into the realm of social regulation—through awareness—and economic regulation, by subsidizing or providing free diagnostic tests.

Data collection and the information on commercial providers, necessary for effective regulation, are typically limited in developing countries. There is often poor awareness of existing regulation amongst commercial providers, and communication of regulatory requirements is often limited (Stenson 1997;Kumaranayake 2000). There is also little evidence of the involvement of commercial sector organizations or representatives of professional associations in regulatory processes. Whilst there is a common view that the commercial sector provides a better quality of health care, the evidence on this remains unclear, and significant problems with quality, opportunistic behaviour, and malpractice in the commercial sector have been observed (Patouillard et al. 2007; Bloom et al. 2009).

Economic regulation seeks to control variables such as price, quantity, quality, and competition in market transactions. The quality dimension in this equation needs further clarification. It is fostered by minimum standards of service delivery. Standardization, as we have explained earlier, belongs to the social regulation domain. Achieving the latter is riddled with complexities and challenges. There are few examples in the literature of price control or effective policies to manage competition between commercial providers or to develop consumer protection laws. India has introduced such an act, The Consumer Protection Act 1986, but this has been poorly implemented, with little response to complaints by consumers against health care providers (Bhat 1999). Below par implementation leaves behind a lot of questions and has a negative influence on future plans too when it comes to a sector as onerous and demanding as health.

Historically, medical professionals and their associations have been self-regulating (Jacobson 2001). In developing countries, medical professionals commonly dominate ministries and departments of health and may themselves be instrumental in the designing of health policy and healthcare regulation. The regulation of the medical profession is difficult and generally requires self-regulation through the involvement of medical associations (WHO 2000). The main regulatory instruments used by the state are licensing and registration of professionals. The quality of education, training, and continued professional development of doctors is poorly monitored and generally delegated to professional associations. Nevertheless, medical associations can play an important role in controlling standards and quality, implementing professional standards, codes of conduct, medical ethics, accreditation, and continued professional development, all of which can influence the behaviour and quality of providers. However, much better results can be acquired by independent regulating organizations with well-defined mandates, underpinned by legislation. The examples in this context are the Punjab Healthcare Commission in Pakistan and the Private Health Services Regulatory Council in Sri Lanka.

The combination of poor government salaries and the growth of the commercial sector has increased the preference of medical and allied health professionals to move into private hospital facilities and clinics (WHO 2000). Private providers, therefore, increasingly compete with the public sector for both human resources and patients, and in many countries, the same providers move between public and private practice. Private practice amongst public sector health workers is very high in developing countries with low regulation (Kiwanuka et al. 2011). This has an impact on equity, efficiency, and availability of services in public facilities and is a considerable problem in South Asia (Dussault 2008). The impact of dual practice depends on the regulatory framework. This, basically, falls in the domain of economic regulation, in which South Asian learning curves are clearly underdeveloped. Monitoring for regulation in South Asia capacity is usually inconsistent and does not augur well for effective regulation. Questions are raised about the capacity regarding operational efficiency and the competence of officers responsible for regulation and quality (Momina et al. 2016). Monitoring, as a component of regulation, in the maternal and reproductive healthcare area is more challenging and needs greater capacity and perseverance. Pakistan and India, being federations, have had multilayered governance structures which in turn has led to complications for regulation in the health sector.

Regulatory organizations can start working at cross purposes, and this happens primarily when regulation is left to professional associations instead of regulatory authorities or commissions, as has happened in India (Peters and Muraleedharan 2008). Professional associations do tend to promote or safeguard narrow professional, cliquish, or even parochial interests. The private stakeholders have an aversion to regulation. Whatever its origins, orientation, or dispensation, regulation in the health sector is dominated by the state. The private sector resents this, in particular, regulation which has an economic and profit curtailing focus. We also need to consider that transaction costs can get out of hand. The maternal health area is multidimensional and has several cross-cutting themes associated with it. Enforcement costs of regulation inevitably go up in such a situation, thus giving rise to the question of perceived benefits of costly enforcement of health regulation in resource-poor countries (Ensor and Weinzierl 2007). Cost of regulation includes, but is not limited due to its transactive nature, to the cost of (i) data collection, (i) inspection, and (iii) monitoring. Regulation requires skilled personnel and dedicated departments or units, appropriately equipped to enforce rules (Akhtar 2011). Looking at the entire gamut of maternal healthcare interventions, already enlisted lucidly in our discourse above, it can be safely inferred that costs of regulatory enforcement can only be ignored at our own peril.

Maternal and reproductive health has cross-sectoral linkages with education and human development and also poverty reduction. These linkages, though not germane to regulation, need to be understood and factored in the purposes of clarity and precision. Without having developed the requisite and sufficient capacity, venturing into health regulation is fraught with serious risks and bound to cause major failures. Ambitious regulatory efforts can also fall short or underachieve because of the lack of resources to implement them. In particular, as we move to the higher-end service delivery, like that in the tertiary care hospitals, efforts for the accreditation of public and private hospitals are clearly cost-intensive. Nandraj cites a pertinent example in this case from India in which lack of resources to finance the accreditation system became the obstacle in its implementation, despite mass support for it from the public and other stakeholders (Nandraj et al. 2001). Lack of communication about regulation itself is pervasive, and most practitioners have little or no knowledge about its rationale. Fudged or engineered data has been a perpetual problem which has created severe constraints for the already demanding process of regulation. Maternal mortality rates (MMR) and contraceptive prevalence rates (CPR) are questioned quite often in South Asia due to the lack of veracity historically. Geographical disparities and variations in terms of capacity both on providers and purchasers side across regions of South Asia are also a major issue that has beset traditional regulation. The capacity at bigger and main urban centres cannot be equated with that in the peripheral towns and more so with villages. Within South Asia, the disparities have urban and rural dimensions.

The institutions of the state, no matter how well-equipped they may be, are beset with issues of organizational and management capacity in health sector regulation. And when it comes to the maternal and reproductive health sub-sectors, the capacity deficit exacerbates as the number of providers from the market, and the civil society is much bigger. This is central to the very theme and imperatives of regulation. Any regulatory effort devoid of independence and operational autonomy will be misleading and self-deluding and will underachieve inevitably. Nunes, Rego, and Brandao in their paper evaluated if independent healthcare regulation is a significant tool with respect to the creation of fair processes for setting desirable limits to health care. They argue that in publicly financed healthcare systems, independent regulation is an important instrument to ensure fair and reasonable procedures of prioritizing services (Nunes et al. 2009). In accordance with the principle of public accountability, independent regulatory agencies are particularly well-suited to accomplish the onerous mandate of regulation. The authors conclude by emphasizing the "social task" of assuring that rationales of "limit-setting decisions" are clearly and tangibly recorded so as to be accessible to the public.

Most regulation globally has tended to focus on controlling the entry of health professionals and organizations into the market through registration and licensing (Doherty 2015). Most countries have not been able to develop sufficient legislation or other regulatory measures to control behaviour by private providers in terms of coverage, quality, distribution, and price and tend to rely on self-regulation primarily backed up by sanctions imposed by health professional councils against the more extreme cases of inappropriate practice. This, for obvious reasons, is a recipe for underperformance. Whilst several developing countries have ventured into updating and improving their legislations, in most cases, the progress and the remaining problems are much the same as identified years ago (Doherty 2015).

Given the limitations of business-as-usual models, a newer and more inclusive approach, with innovations, is obviously called for. A few workable and tested approaches will be discussed in the rest of this section. Responsive regulation attempts to move beyond the ideological debate that views market and state relations as a dichotomy (Ayres and Braithwaite 1995). This approach is based on an understanding that the best regulatory strategies depend essentially on context, regulatory culture, and history. It accepts that, with the emergence of new actors in regulation and policy, command and control models of regulation have become questionable if not outright redundant. More importantly, this school of thought believes that single regulatory instruments are seldom effective and that clearly different approaches are needed (Healy and Braithwaite 2006). It is an approach that values trust, transparency, and professionalism. It aims to reduce the polarized choice between punishment and persuasion, with punishment applying more to anti-quackery.

Braithwaite has argued that developing countries are "more lacking in all the capacities" required to make responsive regulation work well compared to the developed and wealthy economies (Healy and Braithwaite 2006). Braithwaite asserts that two new strategies are needed for networked governance to address these capacity deficits, in which governance efforts are not top-down, but collaborative (Healy and Braithwaite 2006). One is based on the pyramidal escalation of network branching, and the second is legislating for *qui tam* actions or bounty hunting by whistle-blowers. The crucial difference between the old "Command and Control" view is that governments are increasingly "steering (instead of rowing)" and are seeking flexible, participatory, and devolved forms of regulation. In another vein, decentralized regulation is a reaction to the statist, centralized model. It expands the regulatory effort beyond the state and makes it more inclusive. It does not have a predilection for control; rather, it aims to "influence" the behaviour of actors. It complements decentralized regulation most appropriately. Consultation with civil society networks or consumer groups is advised to the health providers. It is dubbed as the move away from traditional reactive model rooted in "minimum standards", where we only act when something goes wrong and are interested in things which are "illegal" (Dickson 2016).

Maternal and child health needs all forms of regulation in some modicum. The "Command and Control" form is useful in anti-quackery efforts, whereas "meta-regulation" and "self-regulation" can be of immense utility in hospitals and maternal healthcare centres. Ultimately, South Asia requires a responsive regulation, which may opt for a range of regulatory options. The pyramid model recommended by Healy and Braithwaite is an attempt to solve the puzzle as to when to persuade and when to punish (Healy and Braithwaite 2006). A regulator begins with persuasion, through a dialogue-based approach for securing compliance with a just rule or standard and by invoking informal rewards rather than sanctions. The persuasion approach is considered a "soft approach," which has modest expectations attached to it, especially in a developing country context. Thus, at times, more demanding strategies are invoked, through which everyone is informed and conscious that non-compliance may result in alternative strategies.

Persistent infractions or infringements may eventually elicit repeat inspections and public disclosure of failure to meet standards, in which case referral to support services or mentoring should be offered and employed. Continued and serious breaches of the regulatory guidelines may incur financial penalties, leading to activities and interventions being curtailed or disbanded. Deregistration of a doctor or a medic, license removal or suspension, and outright closure of the hospital or health facility are cited as last resorts and signal the failure of both parties to ensure that the public is well served. Some argue that the private health sector understands only the "bottom line" profit and therefore must be punished for violations or infringements when their performance is subjected to regulation. Others assert that the private sector can be persuaded. Both the positions, the truth is, are valid depending on the context and prevailing conditions. Neither consistent punishment nor consistent persuasion has proven effective over the long term. Consistent punishment is too costly, and consistent cajoling of the incorrigibly unethical or incompetent is naïve. It has also been noted with concern that regulators who were consistently "tolerant and understanding" ended up increasing non-compliance (Makkai and Braithwaite 1994). This, inevitably, is also a common practice in developing countries and in South Asia.

Maternal health is an area of specialization that needs a very high level of diligence and commitment. The maternal mortality figures across the South Asian countries, excluding Sri Lanka, are a telltale of the struggle that was encountered or is being encountered in turning the situation around. Different facets of maternal health care require different interventions and different levels of effort. The poignancy and pathos attached with maternal health indicators draw governments a lot of flak and criticism. The most noticeable fact to have emerged in health sectors of several developing countries and pretty much all the South Asian countries is that of co-production. Co-production has been acknowledged as a reality and has assumed the dimensions of a need. Co-production is the provision of public services, broadly defined to include regulation, through an institutionalized, long-term relationship between state agencies and organized groups of citizens, where both make substantial resource contributions. It is in keeping with the paradigm of "governance". Governance is the paradigmatic framework wherein the triangle for development and public policy gets completed—the state at the apex, the market, and the civil society. Co-production, for obvious reasons, requires a special effort when it comes to health regulation. Decentralized regulation involves a shift away from the state as the sole regulator. It expands regulatory activities to actors and measures beyond the state and "delimits" regulation as an act of control to a range of activities and mechanisms that can influence the behaviour of actors (Black 2002).

Proponents of decentralized regulation identify reasons why traditional regulation systems have failed in the health sector, which will be discussed in the rest of this section (Akhtar 2011). The collapse of the public-private distinction presents a real challenge for regulation because it calls into question the very role of formal authorities. Within an overlapping public-private system, hybrid organizations and networks combine governmental and non-governmental actors in different manners. In this environment, regulation becomes a product of activity conducted by these mixed systems. This situation has led to the emergence of co-regulation as a strategic choice. Fragmentation of knowledge, power, and control goes further and deeper than mere information asymmetry (Akhtar 2011). It goes without saying that no single actor can ever have the knowledge or information required to solve complex problems. Therefore, no single actor can employ the instruments necessary to regulate. Fragmentation of power means that different actors hold different levels and degrees of power, and the government does not have a monopoly on power. Instead, power is dispersed amongst the state and other actors in the triangular relationship, with the state at the apex and the other two sides of the triangle being occupied by the market (commercial sector) and the civil society.

The health system is complex, to the extent that it can befuddle people with its intricacies. The process of interaction between the various components and actors is dynamic and imperfectly understood. Actors have diverse goals, norms, and power, and they harbour their own intentions (Akhtar 2011). This complexity needs to be torn down. Regulation can help to bring in the elusive clarity, which is so very vital for improving the state of affairs in the critical and highly sensitive area of maternal health. Actors will continue to behave as they wish in the absence of intervention. Actors and systems are therefore often self-regulating (Akhtar 2011). Interventions will have good and bad unintended effects, and no single actor can dominate the regulatory process because of the autonomy of the other actors. This is how delicately the health system is structured. Furthermore, actors and systems do have the capacity to regulate themselves competently enough, and this capacity should be harnessed to be made more effective.

The decentralized approach to regulation allows for the non-state actors, networks, and the health sector associations to interact in dual roles as regulators and the regulated. They are involved in co-producing regulation that may not be bureaucratic instruments aimed at control over economic and social activities, but milder and subtler ways of organizing and exchanging information to influence behaviour and regulatory outcomes. Decentralized regulation, therefore, becomes a strategic approach that can be utilized by the state to implement a range of regulatory strategies. Akhtar (2011), however, maintains that it does not need to be the sole agent working on regulation, detecting deviations and violations and enforcing rules. The health sector has its own peculiarities: maternal health even more so. We need to imbibe constructs from the typology of public policy too. One of the types of public policy is regulatory policy. It is further classified into competitive regulatory policy and protective regulatory policy. Both these categories can assist in regulating the maternal health sub-sector very well. Competitive regulatory policy is designed to limit the provision of goods and services to a few designated deliverers, who are chosen from a larger number of competing potential deliverers.

Protective regulatory policies seek to protect the public and consumers from market problems, such as deceptive advertising (from quacks, for instance), faulty products (spurious drugs), or negative externalities (e.g. pollution). There are several examples from South Asian countries with regard to registration of healthcare professionals. Putting barriers to enter a profession is like raising a bar with a view to ensuring the availability of skilled workforce and preventing the incidence of quackery. This becomes even more sensitive given the mandate and dimensions of maternal health care and the dependency of South Asian women on community providers. Thus, for the region, the registration of community midwives and community health workers is critical. The effort at registration and licensing of hospitals through the vehicle of Minimum Service Delivery Standards (MSDS) has been a good start and has taken the health sector regulation to a much higher level in the developed world. This effort needs to be documented assiduously and tracked for uniformity across all the spaces of South Asia to ensure comprehensive regulatory policy.

9.4 Maternal and Reproductive Health: Situation Analysis and Regulation Needs

Maternal and reproductive health statistics of South Asian countries make interesting but mostly perturbing reading. Sri Lanka has been the outlier in many respects, having traditionally done well for maternal health services. Data from Tables 9.1 and 9.2 tells us that there is critical need to reduce MMR and increase CPR. This requires monitoring and regulation of antenatal care deliveries conducted at health facilities, deliveries conducted by skilled birth attendants (SBAs), and improved postnatal care. Also, important to be kept under observation are the limitation in services, such as: (i) outreach services for family planning services and (ii) advocacy and behaviour change communication material. This multipronged regulation effort requires an array of stakeholders and not just state actors alone. We can read

Table 9.1 Maternal mortality rates (MMR) and contraception prevalence rates (CPR) for South Asian countries

Country	MMR	CPR
Pakistan	178	34%
India	174	50%
Bangladesh	176	62%
Sri Lanka	30	65%
Nepal	258	53%

Source: Data for this table has been retrieved from publically available data sets of the Demographic Health Surveys and Family Health Surveys of Pakistan (2017–2018)

Table 9.2 Maternal health indicators for South Asian countries

Country	Births at health facility	Deliveries conducted by SBAs	Antenatal care	Postnatal care
Pakistan	66%	69%	86%	62%
India	79%	85.1%	84%	67.5%
Nepal	57%	42%	84%	36%
Bangladesh	37%	58%	64%	57%
Sri Lanka	99.5%	99.5%	99%	99%

Source: Data for this table has been retrieved from publically available data sets of the Demographic Health Surveys and Family Health Surveys of Pakistan (2017–2018)

from Table 9.1 that the maternal mortality rate (MMR) for South Asian states is very high. Nepal, Pakistan, Bangladesh, and India lead the dismal statistics by 258, 178, 176, and 174 maternal deaths per 100,000 live births, respectively. Contraception prevalence rates (CPR) are low in Pakistan, India, and Nepal, at 34%, 50%, and 53%, respectively.

Table 9.2 helps to explain both critical issues of high MMR and low CPR, with respect to variables of birth at healthcare centres, delivery by skilled birth attendants, and antenatal and postnatal health care. We can read that Sri Lanka's success in reducing MMR is mainly due to very high incidence of births at healthcare centres, delivery by skilled birth attendants, and antenatal and postnatal health care access. Conversely, Bangladesh, Nepal, and Pakistan, at 37%, 57%, and 66%, respectively, have fewer women delivering at a healthcare facility and more women delivering in their homes.

For Tables 9.3, 9.4, and 9.5, we have used publically available health data sets for women of South Asia. Data collected in Demographic and Health Surveys (DHS) includes samples across Bangladesh, India, and Pakistan of women of reproductive ages, from 15 to 49 years. We were unable to analyze data from other South Asian states due to lack of data all together or lack of available date in recent years. In Table 9.3, we present chi-square associations between possession of health card for child vaccination and dependent socio-demographic and health behaviour variables of Bangladeshi women. Though our aim in this analysis was to keep health insurance as a dependent variable, this variable was missing in the Bangladesh DHS. This may imply that a significant number of women do not have health insurance in Bangladesh, as suggested by other literature (Joarder et al. 2019). Also included in the missing variable list, in our analysis for India and Pakistan, are house and land ownership. The sample of Bangladesh women who had a health card for child immunization was N = 6,680, of which N = 422 "do not have a health card" and N = 6,258 "have a health card".

Majority of sampled women in Bangladesh are from the poor or middle class (59.0%), belong to the rural areas (67.6%), and are not working (73.0%). Demographically, it is important that the public healthcare system is geared to support the disadvantaged women of Bangladesh. Majority of women visited a prenatal doctor (58.9%), but majority also delivered their baby at home (60.0%). The results imply that possibly after women have been told by trained practitioners that their

Table 9.3 Chi-square associations between possession of health card for child vaccination and dependent variables of Bangladeshi women of reproductive age, N = 6680; do not have a health card (HC) = 422; has or had a health card (HC) = 6258

Variable		Total women	No HC	With HC	Chi square	P value
Age in 5-year groups	15–19	15.3%	1.2%	14.2%	31.03	0.029
	20–24	33.1%	2.0%	31.1%		
	25–29	27.5%	1.6%	25.9%		
	30–34	15.8%	0.9%	14.9%		
	35–39	6.3%	0.4%	5.9%		
	40–44	1.5%	0.1%	1.4%		
	45–49	0.4%	0.1%	0.4%		
		100.0%	6.3%	93.7%		
Type of place of residence	Urban	32.4%	1.5%	30.9%	41.23	0.000
	Rural	67.6%	4.8%	62.8%		
		100.0%	6.3%	93.7%		
Region	Barisal	12.0%	0.5%	11.5%	246.674	0.000
	Chittagong	18.7%	1.3%	17.4%		
	Dhaka	17.9%	0.6%	17.3%		
	Khulna	11.3%	0.6%	10.7%		
	Rajshahi	12.5%	0.6%	12.0%		
	Rangpur	12.8%	0.4%	12.4%		
	Sylhet	14.7%	2.2%	12.5%		
		100.0%	6.3%	93.7%		
Highest educational level	No education	15.0%	1.8%	13.1%	137.12	0.000
	Primary	27.2%	1.9%	25.3%		
	Secondary	46.7%	2.1%	44.6%		
	Higher	11.2%	0.5%	10.7%		
		100.0%	6.3%	93.7%		
Wealth index	Poorest	20.8%	2.1%	18.7%	122.70	0.000
	Poorer	18.7%	1.4%	17.3%		
	Middle	19.5%	1.2%	18.3%		
	Richer	20.7%	1.0%	19.6%		
	Richest	20.3%	0.6%	19.7%		
		100.0%	6.3%	93.7%		
Occupation	Not working	73.0%	4.8%	68.2%	82.6	0.000
	Professional/technical/managerial	2.2%	0.1%	2.1%		
	Sales	1.9%	0.1%	1.8%		
	Agricultural – self employed	0.6%	0.0%	0.5%		
	Agricultural – employee	11.3%	0.6%	10.7%		
	Household and domestic	1.6%	0.2%	1.5%		

(continued)

Table 9.3 (continued)

Variable		Total women	No HC	With HC	Chi square	P value
	Services	2.1%	0.2%	1.9%		
	Skilled manual	7.3%	0.3%	7.1%		
	Unskilled manual	0.0%	0.0%	0.0%		
		100.0%	6.3%	93.7%		
Number of children	1–2	68.6%	3.4%	65.2%	143.72	0.000
	3 or more	31.4%	3.0%	28.5%		
		100.0%	6.3%	93.7%		
Prenatal: doctor	No	41.1%	4.5%	36.6%	42.72	0.000
	Yes	58.9%	3.6%	55.3%		
		100.0%	8.1%	91.9%		
Place of delivery	Respondent's home	60.0%	5.7%	54.3%	58.22	0.004
	Public hospital	3.6%	0.2%	3.4%		
	District hospital	3.1%	0.3%	2.7%		
	Maternal and child welfare centre	2.8%	0.1%	2.7%		
	Upazila health complex	3.6%	0.2%	3.4%		
	Upazila health and family welfare centre	0.5%	0.0%	0.4%		
	Other public sector	0.0%	0.0%	0.0%		
	Community clinic	0.0%	0.0%	0.0%		
	Private hospital/clinic	23.2%	1.3%	22.0%		
	NGO static clinic	2.8%	0.3%	2.5%		
	Other NGO sector	0.2%	0.0%	0.2%		
	Other	0.1%	0.0%	0.1%		
		100.0%	8.2%	91.8%		
Size of child at birth	Very large	2.2%	0.0%	2.2%	19.89	0.069
	Larger than average	10.8%	0.8%	10.1%		
	Average	67.7%	5.1%	62.5%		
	Smaller than average	12.9%	1.5%	11.5%		
	Very small	6.3%	0.7%	5.6%		
		100.0%	8.1%	91.9%		

Source: Data for this table has been retrieved from the publically available data sets of the Demographic Health Survey of Bangladesh (2014–2015)

pregnancy is normal, they do not opt for institutional deliveries. Nearly all mothers of Bangladesh indicated that their child was average or small at birth (87.0%), implying that there is great need for regulation for prenatal health of the mother to reduce the incidence of small size at birth and also child stunting in the country. We found that all chi-square results were significant, implying that all these variables of socio-demographic and health indicators have a significant association with having a health card in women of Bangladesh.

Table 9.4 Chi-square associations between health insurance and dependent variables of Indian women of reproductive age, N = 699,686; not covered by Health Insurance (HI) = 574,718; covered by Health Insurance (HI) = 124,968

Variable		Total	No HI	With HI	Chi square	P value
Age in 5-year groups	15–19	17.8%	15.1%	2.7%	3900.15	0.000
	20–24	17.6%	15.0%	2.5%		
	25–29	16.4%	13.8%	2.7%		
	30–34	13.9%	11.3%	2.6%		
	35–39	12.9%	10.3%	2.6%		
	40–44	11.0%	8.6%	2.3%		
	45–49	10.4%	8.0%	2.4%		
		100.0%	82.1%	17.9%		
Type of place of residence	Urban	29.3%	24.4%	4.9%	298.61	0.000
	Rural	70.7%	57.7%	13.0%		
		100.0%	82.1%	17.9%		
State	Andaman and Nicobar Islands	0.4%	0.4%	0.0%	161846.11	0.000
	Andhra Pradesh	1.5%	0.4%	1.0%		
	Arunachal Pradesh	2.0%	0.9%	1.1%		
	Assam	4.1%	3.9%	0.2%		
	Bihar	6.5%	6.0%	0.5%		
	Chandigarh	0.1%	0.1%	0.0%		
	Chhattisgarh	3.6%	1.2%	2.4%		
	Dadra and Nagar Haveli	0.1%	0.1%	0.0%		
	Daman and Diu	0.2%	0.2%	0.0%		
	Goa	0.2%	0.2%	0.0%		
	Gujarat	3.3%	2.7%	0.6%		
	Haryana	3.1%	3.0%	0.1%		
	Himachal Pradesh	1.4%	1.2%	0.2%		
	Jammu and Kashmir	3.4%	3.4%	0.0%		
	Jharkhand	4.2%	3.8%	0.3%		
	Karnataka	3.8%	2.9%	0.9%		
	Kerala	1.6%	0.9%	0.7%		
	Lakshadweep	0.2%	0.2%	0.0%		
	Madhya Pradesh	9.0%	7.9%	1.1%		
	Maharashtra	4.2%	3.9%	0.3%		
	Manipur	1.9%	1.9%	0.0%		
	Meghalaya	1.3%	0.9%	0.4%		
	Mizoram	1.8%	1.4%	0.4%		
	Nagaland	1.5%	1.5%	0.0%		
	Delhi	0.8%	0.8%	0.1%		
	Odisha	4.8%	2.9%	1.9%		
	Puducherry	0.6%	0.5%	0.1%		

(continued)

Table 9.4 (continued)

Variable		Total	No HI	With HI	Chi square	P value
	Punjab	2.8%	2.5%	0.3%		
	Rajasthan	6.0%	5.3%	0.7%		
	Sikkim	0.8%	0.6%	0.2%		
	Tamil Nadu	4.1%	2.4%	1.7%		
	Tripura	0.7%	0.3%	0.4%		
	Uttar Pradesh	14.0%	13.6%	0.4%		
	Uttarakhand	2.5%	2.2%	0.3%		
	West Bengal	2.5%	1.9%	0.7%		
	Telangana	1.1%	0.4%	0.7%		
		100.0%	82.1%	17.9%		
Highest educational level	No education	28.1%	23.2%	4.9%	294.86	0.000
	Primary	12.6%	10.1%	2.5%		
	Secondary	47.9%	39.4%	8.5%		
	Higher	11.4%	9.4%	2.0%		
		100.0%	82.1%	17.9%		
Wealth index	Poorest	19.0%	15.8%	3.3%	1003.44	0.000
	Poorer	21.4%	17.4%	3.9%		
	Middle	21.0%	16.9%	4.1%		
	Richer	19.8%	16.2%	3.6%		
	Richest	18.8%	15.9%	2.9%		
		100.0%	82.1%	17.9%		
Occupation	Not in workforce/no occupation	69.6%	10.2%	2.0%	294.86	0.000
	Professional/technical/ managerial	2.8%	0.4%	0.1%		
	Clerical	0.4%	0.0%	0.0%		
	Sales	1.5%	0.2%	0.1%		
	Agricultural	15.1%	2.0%	0.6%		
	Services/household and domestic	3.3%	0.4%	0.2%		
	Manual – skilled and unskilled	6.2%	0.8%	0.3%		
	Don't know	1.1%	0.2%	0.0%		
		100.0%	14.2%	3.2%		
Total children	None	31.9%	26.8%	5.1%	2072.87	0.000
	1–3	36.0%	29.0%	7.0%		
	3 or more	32.2%	26.3%	5.8%		
		100.0%	82.1%	17.9%		
Household has electricity	No	10.4%	9.3%	1.1%	3225.96	0.000
	Yes	86.4%	70.1%	16.3%		
	Not a de jure resident	3.2%	2.8%	0.4%		
		100.0%	82.1%	17.9%		

(continued)

Table 9.4 (continued)

Variable		Total	No HI	With HI	Chi square	P value
Owns a house alone or jointly	Does not own	61.2%	8.8%	1.9%	1023.08	0.000
	Alone only	9.4%	1.2%	0.5%		
	Jointly only	17.0%	2.4%	0.5%		
	Both alone and jointly	12.4%	1.8%	0.3%		
		100.0%	14.2%	3.2%		
Owns land alone or jointly	Does not own	69.8%	10.0%	2.2%	725.33	0.000
	Alone only	6.5%	0.8%	0.3%		
	Jointly only	13.6%	1.9%	0.4%		
	Both alone and jointly	10.1%	1.5%	0.3%		
		100.0%	14.2%	3.2%		
Prenatal: doctor	No	45.5%	11.0%	1.5%	932.87	0.000
	Yes	54.5%	12.4%	2.5%		
		100.0%	23.3%	3.9%		
Place of delivery	Respondent's home	19.8%	4.7%	0.7%	404.92	0.000
	Other home	0.2%	0.1%	0.0%		
	Parents' Home	2.1%	0.5%	0.1%		
	Public: Govt./Municipal Hospital	25.0%	5.8%	1.1%		
	Public: Govt. Dispensary	1.7%	0.4%	0.1%		
	Public: UHC/UHP/ UFWC	1.5%	0.4%	0.1%		
	Public: Rural Hospital	18.5%	4.3%	0.7%		
	Public: PHC/Additional PHC	7.3%	1.7%	0.3%		
	Public: Sub-Centre	1.2%	0.3%	0.1%		
	Other Public Sector Facility	0.1%	0.0%	0.0%		
	Private: Hospital /Clinic	21.3%	5.0%	0.8%		
	Other Private Sector Facility	0.5%	0.1%	0.0%		
	NGO or Trust Hospital/ Clinic	0.5%	0.1%	0.0%		
	Other	0.2%	0.1%	0.0%		
		100.0%	23.3%	3.9%		
Size of child at birth	Very large	5.1%	1.2%	0.2%	327.83	0.000
	Larger than average	12.4%	2.8%	0.6%		
	Average	68.4%	16.0%	2.6%		
	Smaller than average	9.0%	2.1%	0.3%		
	Very small	2.9%	0.7%	0.1%		
	Don't know	2.1%	0.5%	0.1%		

(continued)

Table 9.4 (continued)

Variable		Total	No HI	With HI	Chi square	P value
		100.0%	23.3%	3.9%		

Source: Data for this table has been retrieved from the publically available data set of the Demographic Health Survey of India (2015–2016)

In Table 9.4, we present the chi-square associations between health insurance and dependent socio-demographic and health behaviour variables of Indian women. The sample of women from India is *N* = 699,686, of which *N* = 574,718 are "not covered by health insurance" and *N* = 124,968 are "covered by health insurance. Findings confirm that majority women of India are not covered by health insurance and instead rely on out-of-pocket finances for health. Majority of women are from the poor or middle class (61.4%), belong to the rural areas (70.7%), and are not working (69.6%). Majority of women do not own houses (61.2%) or land (69.8%), and results imply a major problem in ownership and empowerment for women in the country. Like in Bangladesh, the Indian healthcare infrastructure and policy need to be oriented to support majority disadvantaged women in the country. India is a large country with great provincial and ethnic diversity, and the equity of health-care services for women across different states must also be a major consideration for policymakers. Only 54.5% of women have taken assistance from a trained doctor during prenatal period, but unlike Bangladesh, fewer Indian women are delivering their child at home (22.1%). A near majority of women feel their child was of average or small size at birth (80.3%). All chi-square results were highly significant, suggesting that having or not having health insurance is associated with socio-demographic and health characteristics in mothers.

Table 9.5 presents chi-square associations between health insurance and dependent socio-demographic and health behaviour variables of Pakistani women. The sample for the Pakistan DHS is N = 15,066, with N = 14,748 "not covered by health insurance" and N = 318 "covered by health insurance". Findings confirm dismal figures of nearly all women being deprived of health insurance. Majority of the sample belong to the poor or middle class (60.4%), are from rural areas (51.9%), and are not working (84.6%). Nearly all women do not own houses or land at 97.0% and 98.0%, respectively. Our findings imply there is great need to improve state-level awareness for property rights of women and also legally enforce property rights. The statistics suggest that possibly religious laws are not being followed with regard to wealth distribution amongst daughters, wives, and widows. Compared to Bangladesh and India, majority women of Pakistan are not educated (50.6%), and majority have three or more children (58.6%). The implications are that in Pakistan there is critical need for increasing educational opportunities for women and also improving family planning policies to control population explosion. A considerable number of women at 20.5% do not visit a licensed doctor during the prenatal period and 32.8% of women deliver their children in homes. Nearly all women indicated that their child was of either average of small size when born (91.8%).

Table 9.5 Chi-square associations between health insurance and dependent variables of Pakistani women of reproductive age, N = 15,066; not covered by Health Insurance (HI) = 318; covered by Health Insurance (HI) = 14,748

Variable		Total	No HI	With HI	Chi square	P value
Age in 5-year groups	15–19	4.8%	4.8%	0.0%	55.66	0.000
	20–24	14.7%	14.6%	0.1%		
	25–29	20.9%	20.5%	0.3%		
	30–34	18.9%	18.4%	0.5%		
	35–39	18.2%	17.6%	0.6%		
	40–44	12.1%	11.7%	0.4%		
	45–49	10.4%	10.1%	0.3%		
		100.0%	97.9%	2.1%		
Type of place of residence	Urban	48.1%	47.0%	1.2%	7.98	0.005
	Rural	51.9%	50.9%	0.9%		
		100.0%	97.9%	2.1%		
Region	Punjab	22.6%	22.2%	0.3%	257.66	0.000
	Sindh	18.2%	18.0%	0.1%		
	KPK	15.8%	15.2%	0.6%		
	Balochistan	11.4%	11.4%	0.1%		
	GB	6.5%	6.0%	0.5%		
	ICT	7.4%	7.1%	0.2%		
	AJK	11.4%	11.2%	0.2%		
	FATA	6.7%	6.7%	0.0%		
		100.0%	97.9%	2.1%		
Highest educational level	No education	50.6%	49.9%	0.7%	151.2	0.000
	Primary	14.0%	13.7%	0.2%		
	Secondary	20.8%	20.5%	0.3%		
	Higher	14.6%	13.8%	0.8%		
		100.0%	97.9%	2.1%		
Wealth index combined	Poorest	19.2%	18.9%	0.2%	40.35	0.000
	Poorer	21.5%	21.1%	0.4%		
	Middle	19.7%	19.3%	0.4%		
	Richer	19.1%	18.7%	0.4%		
	Richest	20.5%	19.8%	0.7%		
		100.0%	97.9%	2.1%		
Occupation	Not working	84.6%	83.1%	1.5%	283.05	0.000
	Professional/technical/ managerial	3.4%	3.0%	0.4%		
	Clerical	0.1%	0.1%	0.0%		
	Sales	0.5%	0.5%	0.0%		
	Agricultural— self employed	3.4%	3.4%	0.0%		

(continued)

Table 9.5 (continued)

Variable		Total	No HI	With HI	Chi square	P value
	Services	1.9%	1.9%	0.0%		
	Skilled manual	5.3%	5.2%	0.0%		
	Unskilled manual	0.8%	0.8%	0.0%		
		100.0%	97.9%	2.1%		
Total children	None	12.9%	12.8%	0.2%	20.19	0.164
	1–2	28.5%	27.9%	0.6%		
	3 or more	58.6%	57.2%	1.4%		
Owns a house alone or jointly	Does not own	97.0%	95.1%	2.0%	21.28	0.000
	Alone only	1.5%	1.5%	0.1%		
	Jointly only	1.3%	1.2%	0.1%		
	Both alone and jointly	0.2%	0.1%	0.0%		
		100.0%	97.9%	2.1%		
Owns land alone or jointly	Does not own	98.0%	96.0%	2.0%	28.29	0.000
	Alone only	1.0%	1.0%	0.1%		
	Jointly only	0.8%	0.8%	0.0%		
	Both alone and jointly	0.1%	0.1%	0.0%		
		100.0%	97.9%	2.1%		
Prenatal: doctor	No	20.5%	20.3%	0.1%	18.03	0.000
	Yes	79.5%	77.8%	1.8%		
		100.0%	98.1%	1.9%		
Place of delivery	Respondent's home	30.3%	29.9%	0.4%	18.81	0.027
	Other home	2.5%	2.5%	0.0%		
	Government hospital	27.7%	27.2%	0.5%		
	Rural health centre	0.6%	0.6%	0.0%		
	Basic health unit	0.6%	0.6%	0.0%		
	Community midwife	0.2%	0.2%	0.0%		
	Other public sector	0.0%	0.0%	0.0%		
	Private hospital/clinic	37.9%	36.9%	1.0%		
	Other private medical sector	0.0%	0.0%	0.0%		
	Other	0.2%	0.2%	0.0%		
		100.0%	98.1%	1.9%		
Size of child at birth	Very large	0.7%	0.7%	0.0%	3.77	0.582
	Larger than average	7.1%	6.9%	0.2%		
	Average	72.9%	71.4%	1.4%		
	Smaller than average	14.2%	14.0%	0.2%		
	Very small	4.7%	4.6%	0.0%		
	Don't know	0.4%	0.4%	0.0%		
		100.0%	98.1%	1.9%		

Source: Data for this table has been retrieved from the publically available data set of the Demographic Health Survey of Pakistan (2017–2018)

9.5 The Nuances and the Major Considerations

We found through the DHS data that maternal and child health indicators are not favourable in South Asia, with implications that there is a shortfall in state regulation. We also know from the earlier discussion in this chapter that the emergence of hybrid public-private and increasingly commercialized health systems requires a new level of thinking about regulatory approaches. A common view is that centralized control through the state is ineffective in regulating the commercial health sector adequately. A decentralized and more calibrated approach to regulation of health care in developing countries can be more effective (Akhtar 2011). A decentralized approach requires, as well as facilitates, commercial health providers and representatives to interact with civil society networks or consumer groups involved in co-regulation. This co-regulation-based approach would have benefits of (i) tackling information gaps, (ii) addressing fragmentation and ungovernability by accepting and adjusting for the interdependencies, (iii) reducing the differences and inequity between public and private, and (iv) negotiated agreement on roles and responsibilities between state and non-state actors.

The decentralized process would focus on a mix of regulatory strategies, such as market approaches, information disclosure, information exchange, standard setting, and consumer protection. It would also facilitate both the competitive and protective regulatory policies, especially the latter. From these strategies, information exchange systems and standard setting should be given priority because reliable information systems that capture the behaviour of market actors are often one of the most costly and complex activities for the state. These types of activities would define a different role and capacity for state authorities than is currently seen in many developing countries, requiring engagement and collaborative forums. Standard setting, as an instrument of regulation, requires deeper involvement of professional and specialist networks. Whilst standard-setting systems exist in many countries, including medical education standards, nursing standards, and medical associations setting standards of clinical care, these are in most of the cases poorly monitored. The question is how to make these standards work through the commercial sector and modify behaviour, particularly in the informal sector. Asking the market or the commercial sector to modify behaviour is mostly a futile effort given the trust and experience deficits. South Asia is a living example and testimony to these realities.

Coordination of the informal sector is difficult and, without incentives or collaborative forums, is unlikely to attract the involvement of informal providers. Incentive approaches come in different forms; the example of accreditation in Mumbai, India, showed that a commercial hospital seized the opportunity to become more competitive by becoming accredited, which sent a signal of quality to consumers. In this case, the lack of financing was the obstacle. But this is where the state can step in and support an enabling environment with collaboration from the commercial sector. Differences between developing countries also need to be considered. With lower institutional capacity, the developing countries are often constrained to seek support from development partners to develop regulatory frameworks. The creation of the Punjab Healthcare Commission in Pakistan was undertaken through a technical assistance grant of the DFID, administered by the ADB under the Punjab Devolved Social Services Programmed.

There is a growing interest and promotion of market-based approaches to the scaling up of healthcare products for the poor, with international organizations such as the International Finance Corporation, World Bank, USAID, non-government organizations (NGOs), and donors, all seeking ways of harnessing the commercial health sector of developing countries. However, efforts to assist country partners in the development of regulatory frameworks and techniques are lagging. The reasons for this are not well documented, but may, in all likelihood, be due to the limited evidence of effective approaches. Evidence also indicates that there is a lack of investment in institutional capacity and seeking different ways of achieving regulatory outcomes. Consequently, the international actor's actively promoting commercialization of the health sector should also provide investment for improved regulatory systems.

Experts believe that the timing of the implementation of regulatory frameworks needs to be closely matched with the growth of the commercial sector. Middle-income countries, which have substantial commercial sectors, may face more barriers to regulation due to the size and fragmentation of the sector. Given the size of the commercial sector, there may be several vested interests resisting the regulatory effort and advancements. Developing countries, on the other hand, may still be in a position to build regulatory capacity and systems that can appropriately regulate growing commercialized health systems before they reach the size of the commercial sector in middle-income countries (Akhtar 2011). Maternal health care is already quite fragmented in South Asian countries. Maternity centres and TBA outlets have registered mushroom growth in the length and breadth of Pakistan, India, and Bangladesh. Regulating such a multitude of centres is an enormous task and needs decentralized and co-regulation.

The regulation mandate in developed countries is shared by state and non-state institutions, which are working together in harmony. It is also evident that consumer groups and consumer information systems are in place. Actors are involved in dynamic processes that keep changing with the changes in the regulatory environment. On the other hand, these conditions are non-existent in developing countries. Therefore, the regulatory challenge is immense. We must also consider the serious consequences of unregulated healthcare markets in developing countries. They include rising inequities, further weakening and hollowing-out of the public sector, opportunistic behaviour, and poor quality or substandard care. Such eventualities undermine health objectives and can damage the weakest and the most vulnerable members of society, specifically women. Regulation of health care in developing countries should always maintain a culture of public interest and gender-based protection. Little empirical research on regulation of health care in developing countries exists. This, obviously, has implications. A great deal more in terms of research needs to provide evidence on low-cost, decentralized approaches that involve a legitimate blend or mix of regulatory strategies by state, non-state, and civil society actors. In addition to this, developing a more nuanced understanding of the institutions and dynamics of existing regulatory systems in the developing countries is of importance.

The growth of commercialized providers and dual practice is driving much of the failure in contemporary developing countries' health systems. This poses serious challenges. More innovative approaches to regulation are needed in order to tackle traditions and legacy of lack of accountability and legitimized corruption in South Asia so that both public and private segments can start working effectively. Typical, run-off-the-mill approaches will not work, as we must consider that South Asian regulatory policies cannot just emulate the West, but must take into consideration traditional, cultural, and ethnic realities of the region. The decentralized approach of engaging with non-state sectors, using information exchange systems and standard setting can provide a useful way of thinking through regulatory reforms and implementing them purposefully. Scholars have suggested, for the Indian context, that the state must provide alternative approaches to regulation of health services, using the multisectoral and collaborative approaches (Peters and Muraleedharan 2008). Poor regulation is a symptom of poor governance essentially and enforces rules that continue to have limited effects and hamper the chances for positive strides in regulatory efforts. Collaborative mechanisms also promote accountability of all stakeholders and providers. Civil society organizations, the media, and provider organizations can play more active roles in disclosing and using information on the use of health resources and the performance as well as genuineness of public and private providers.

9.6 Concluding Recommendations

If the regulation of the existing maternal and reproductive health services in South Asia is improved, it will help to improve the regulatory challenge for gender equity across the health sector. Our analysis leads us to the conclusion that maternal and reproductive health stands to gain from an alteration in cultural assumptions for both competitive and regulatory policies, in the following three ways. Firstly, single regulatory instruments are seldom effective, and different approaches are required and advisable. With this in perspective, we are convinced about the utility of co-regulation in a decentralized manner. Secondly, complementing this will be responsive regulation. The latter needs to be employed strategically and cautiously as getting it right can be difficult. With all this working as a framework, we strongly recommend that the state must stay at the apex of the triangle—calling the shots and not abdicating its regulatory responsibility to the other actors in co-governance.

Lastly, there is great need for regulatory bodies to help raise awareness and provide solutions to reduce mother and child mortality risks, in relation to (I) poverty alleviation and formal sector work participation; (II) rural and urban slum development and provincial equity; (III) educational inclusion and skill development for adult women; (IV) universal health coverage; (V) family planning and population control; (VI) house, land, and asset ownership and inheritance rights; (VII) licensed practitioner visitations and institutional checkups and deliveries; (VIII) use of technology and media for awareness, communication, and health access; (IX) improved licensing and accountability of practitioners to encourage healthcare utilization by licensed providers and also encourage customer demand; (X) improved regulation and accreditation of private providers and price ceilings for diagnostic tests and treatment services; (XI) improved budget allocation for public health sector infrastructure and salaries for human health resources to improved services and retention; (XII) increase recruitment for health regulation workforce and increase budget for regulatory infrastructure in order to improve: (a) data collection, (b) inspection, and (c) monitoring; (XIII) improve regulation for patient safety, hospital/center administration, and error reporting to encourage utilization of services; (XIV) regulation of dual practices of providers between the public and private sector to improve quality services of the public sector; and (XX) specific micro regulation for (a) antenatal care deliveries conducted at health facilities, deliveries conducted by skilled birth attendants, and improved postnatal care, (b) outreach services for family planning services and advocacy and behaviour change communication material, (c) girl child and women's health preconception and under 5 child health to reduce incidence of small size at birth and also child stunting in the country.

References

Aalders, M., & Wilthagen, T. (1997). Moving beyond command-and-control: Reflexivity in the regulation of occupational safety and health and the environment. *Law & Policy, 19*(4), 415–443.

Akhtar, A. (2011). *Health care regulation in low-and middle-income countries: A literature review.* (n.d.). Retrieved fromhttps://www.scribd.com/document/101491382/Health-care-regulation-in-low-and-middle-income-countries-A-literature-review

Ayres, I., & Braithwaite, J. (1995). *Responsive regulation: Transcending the deregulation debate.* New York: Oxford University Press.

Baldwin, B., Cave, M., & Baldwin, R. (1999). *Understanding regulation: Theory, strategy, and practice.* Oxford: Oxford University Press.

Bhat, R. (1999). Characteristics of private medical practice in India: A provider perspective. *Health Policy and Planning, 14*(1), 26–37. https://doi.org/10.1093/heapol/14.1.26.

Black, J. (2002). Regulatory conversations. *Journal of Law and Society, 29*(1), 163–196. https://doi.org/10.1111/1467-6478.00215.

Bloom, G., Kanjilal, B., & Peters, D. (2009). China and India: Bloom and colleagues respond. *Health Affairs, 28*(1), 297–298. https://doi.org/10.1377/hlthaff.28.1.297-a.

Brhlikova, P., Harper, I., Jeffery, R., Rawal, N., Subedi, M., & Santhosh, M. R. (2011). Trust and the regulation of pharmaceuticals: South Asia in a globalised world. *Globalization and Health, 7*(1), 10.

Chakravarty, A., Sahu, A., Biswas, M., Chatterjee, K., & Rath, S. (2015). A study of assessment of patient safety climate in tertiary care hospitals. *Medical Journal Armed Forces India, 71*(2), 152–157.

Cleary, S. M., Molyneux, S., & Gilson, L. (2013). Resources, attitudes and culture: An understanding of the factors that influence the functioning of accountability mechanisms in primary health care settings. *BMC Health Services Research, 13*(1), 320.

Dickson, G. (2016). Health reform in Canada: Enabling perspectives for health leadership. *Healthcare Management Forum, 29*(2), 53–58. https://doi.org/10.1177/0840470416628635.

Doherty, J. E. (2015). Regulating the for-profit private health sector: Lessons from East and Southern Africa. *Health Policy and Planning, 30*(1), i93–i102. https://doi.org/10.1093/heapol/czu111.

Dussault, G. (2008). The health professions and the performance of future health systems in low-income countries: Support or obstacle? *Social Science & Medicine, 66*(10), 2088–2095. https://doi.org/10.1016/j.socscimed.2008.01.035.

Ensor, T., & Weinzierl, S. (2007). Regulating health care in low- and middle-income countries: Broadening the policy response in resource constrained environments. *Social Science & Medicine, 65*(2), 355–366. https://doi.org/10.1016/j.socscimed.2007.03.021.

Healy, J., & Braithwaite, J. (2006). Designing safer health care through responsive regulation. *Medical Journal of Australia, 184*(S10), S56. https://doi.org/10.5694/j.1326-5377.2006.tb00364.x.

Jacobson, P. D. (2001, October 1). *Regulating health care: From self-regulation to self-regulation?* Retrieved from https://muse.jhu.edu/article/15614

Jafree, S. R. (2018). *Women, healthcare, and violence in Pakistan*. Karachi: Oxford University Press.

Jafree, S. R., Zakar, R., Zakar, M. Z., & Fischer, F. (2015). Nurse perceptions of organizational culture and its association with the culture of error reporting: A case of public sector hospitals in Pakistan. *BMC Health Services Research, 16*(1), 3.

Jawaid, S. A. (2014). Punjab Healthcare Commission needs to be supported and strengthened. *Pulse International, 15*(11), 106–108.

Joarder, T., Chaudhury, T. Z., & Mannan, I. (2019). Universal health coverage in Bangladesh: Activities, challenges, and suggestions. *Advances in Public Health, 2019*, 4954095.

Kadaï, A., Sall, F. L., Andriantsara, G., & Perrot, J. (2006). The benefits of setting the ground rules and regulating contracting practices. *Bulletin of the World Health Organization, 84*(11), 897–902. https://doi.org/10.2471/blt.06.030056.

Kiwanuka, S. N., Rutebemberwa, E., Nalwadda, C., Okui, O., Ssengooba, F., Kinengyere, A. A., & Pariyo, G. W. (2011). Interventions to manage dual practice among health workers. *Cochrane Database of Systematic Reviews, 2011*(7), CD008405. https://doi.org/10.1002/14651858.cd008405.pub2.

Kumaranayake, L. (1997). The role of regulation: Influencing private sector activity within health sector reform. *Journal of International Development, 9*(4), 641–649. https://doi.org/10.1002/(sici)1099-1328(199706)9:4<641::aid-jid473>3.0.co;2-8.

Kumaranayake, L. (2000). How do countries regulate the health sector? Evidence from Tanzania and Zimbabwe. *Health Policy and Planning, 15*(4), 357–367. https://doi.org/10.1093/heapol/15.4.357.

Kumaranayake, L., & Watts, C. (2000). HIV/AIDS Prevention and care interventions in Sub-Saharan Africa: An econometric analysis of the costs of scaling-up. *The South African Journal of Economics, 68*(5), 455–467. https://doi.org/10.1111/j.1813-6982.2000.tb01289.x.

Mackintosh, M. (2007). *Planning and market: Strengths, weaknesses and interactions in the provision of less inequitable and better quality health care*. WHO. Retrieved from https://www.who.int/social_determinants/resources/csdh_media/planning_market_regulation_2007_en.pdf

Makkai, T., & Braithwaite, J. (1994). The dialectics of corporate deterrence. *Journal of Research in Crime and Delinquency, 31*(4), 347–373. https://doi.org/10.1177/0022427894031004001.

Manville, C., Hackett, P., Gunashekar, S., & Jones, M. M. (2013). Regulatory cultures and research governance. *Rand Health Quarterly, 3*(1), 5.

Mills, A., Brugha, R., Hanson, K., & McPake, B. (2002). What can be done about the private health sector in low-income countries? *Bulletin of the World Health Organization, 80*, 325–330.

Momina, A.-U., Anwar, S., & Tarin, E. (2016). Punjab Healthcare Commission's regulation of general practitioners of allopathic medicine. *Annals of King Edward Medical University, 22*(1), 63. https://doi.org/10.21649/akemu.v22i1.800.

Nandraj, S., Khot, A., Menon, S., & Ruairí, B. (2001). A stakeholder approach towards hospital accreditation in India. *Health Policy and Planning, 16*(Suppl_2), 70–79. https://doi.org/10.1093/heapol/16.suppl_2.70.
Nunes, R., Rego, G., & Brandão, C. (2009). Healthcare regulation as a tool for public accountability. *Medicine, Health Care and Philosophy, 12*(3), 257–264. https://doi.org/10.1007/s11019-008-9177-4.
Ogus. (1996). Regulation: Legal form and economic theory. *The Modern Law Review, 59*(1), 161–164. https://doi.org/10.5040/9781472559647.
Palmer, N., Strong, L., Wali, A., & Sondorp, E. (2006). Contracting out health services in fragile states. *BMJ, 332*(7543), 718–721. https://doi.org/10.1136/bmj.332.7543.718.
Patouillard, E., Goodman, C. A., Hanson, K. G., & Mills, A. J. (2007). Can working with the private for-profit sector improve utilization of quality health services by the poor? A systematic review of the literature. *International Journal for Equity in Health, 6*(1), 17. https://doi.org/10.1186/1475-9276-6-17.
Peters, D. H., & Muraleedharan, V. (2008). Regulating Indias health services: To what end? What future? *Social Science & Medicine, 66*(10), 2133–2144. https://doi.org/10.1016/j.socscimed.2008.01.037.
Raposo, V. L. (2015). How can Asian countries deal with medical liability and patient compensation. *People: International Journal of Social Sciences, 1*(1), Special Issue.
Roberts, M. J., Roberts, W. J., & Roberts, P. J. (2004). *Getting health reform right: A guide to improving performance and equity*. New York: Oxford University Press.
Sheikh, K., Saligram, P. S., & Hort, K. (2013). What explains regulatory failure? Analysing the architecture of health care regulation in two Indian states. *Health Policy and Planning, 30*(1), 39–55. https://doi.org/10.1093/heapol/czt095.
Stenson, B. (1997). Pharmaceutical regulation in context: The case of Lao Peoples Democratic Republic. *Health Policy and Planning, 12*(4), 329–340. https://doi.org/10.1093/heapol/12.4.329.
Stenson, B., Syhakhang, L., Eriksson, B., & Tomson, G. (2001). Real world pharmacy: Assessing the quality of private pharmacy practice in the Lao People's Democratic Republic. *Social Science & Medicine, 52*(3), 393–404. https://doi.org/10.1016/s0277-9536(00)00142-8.
Teerawattananon, Y., Tangcharoensathien, V., Tantivess, S., & Mills, A. (2003). Health sector regulation in Thailand: Recent progress and the future agenda. *Health Policy, 63*(3), 323–338. https://doi.org/10.1016/s0168-8510(02)00140-9.
Walshe, K. (2003). *Regulating healthcare: A prescription for improvement?* Maidenhead: Open University Press.
Webb, R. K., Currie, M., Morgan, C. A., Williamson, J. A., Mackay, P., Russell, W. J., & Runciman, W. B. (1993). The Australian Incident Monitoring Study: an analysis of 2000 incident reports. *Anaesthesia and intensive care, 21*(5), 520–528.
World Health Organization. (2006). The world health report 2006: working together for health. World Health Organization.
World Health Organization. (2000). The world health report 2000: health systems: improving performance. World Health Organization.

Index

S. R. Jafree (ed.), *The Sociology of South Asian Women's Health*, https://doi.org/10.1007/978-3-030-50204-1

N

The manufacturer's authorised representative in the EU is Springer Nature Customer Service Centre GmbH, Europaplatz 3, 69115 Heidelberg, Germany. If you have any concerns regarding our products, please contact ProductSafety@springernature.com

Printed and bound by CPI Group (UK) Ltd, Croydon, CR0 4YY
30/09/2026
02225651-0005